KINK PHOBIA

Journey Through A Black Woman's Hair

Kink Phobia

Journey Through A Black Woman's Hair

Ella Joyce

FirstPublish
A Division of the Brekel Group, Inc.
control your own destiny

For more information contact:
Ms. Thing Productions, Inc.
18375 Ventura Blvd., Suite 214
Tarzana, CA 91356
email: msthing@mymailstation.com

ISBN
1-929925-86-7

Library of Congress Cataloging in Publication Data
2001094028

Ella Joyce
Kink Phobia

10 9 8 7 6 5 4 3 2 1

FIRSTPUBLISH
A Divison of Brekel Group, Inc.
300 Sunport Ln.
Orlando, FL 32809
407-240-1414
www.firstpublish.com

Dedication

For

Any Sister

who has broken a comb

ACKNOWLEDGMENTS

I would like to acknowledge my Creator for the Divine Inspiration and Courage to write this book.

I would like to thank my sweet husband, Dan Martin, for his devoted support, love, encouragement, and for those private computer lessons.

I would like to acknowledge and thank my parents, Benjamin and Joyce ("Bunnie") Hoye, for their nurturing support and love, as well as my sister, Wandra (for those prayers), and my lovely grandmother, Faye ("Nana") Goode (the treasure in our lives).

I would also like mention a few fantastic braiders in my experience. Sandra ("Sandy") Baldwin - you are phenomenal; Sheila Everette-Hale (a creative genius); and Kelly Taffe (made me a vision of loveliness on my wedding day). Also, I would like to acknowledge a few of my "sisters-of-the-nap". Sisters who personally encouraged and inspired me along the way to write this book, and a few who are proudly sporting their own very kinky curls, naps, twists, and locks: Lammia Tefnut, Chiquita Ross-Glover, Diane Williams, Janice Johnson, Janet Smollett (and family), T'Keyah Crystal Keyman, Margo and Amber Moorer, Joyce Lawson, Denise ("Nesie") Gonzalvez, Valerie Kagel, Brenda Joyce, and Lynne Marie Brown.

I would also like to acknowledge anyone who mentored me in any way with my first publishing venture, as well as my fellow artists whose encouraging comments and genuine enthusiasm gave me insight, courage and support.

CONTENTS

Preface

SISTERS, what are we gonna do 'bout our hair?

Well, that is what this book is about. I'm talking to those of us who are woolly at the root. Woolly to me suggests spongy soft textures, like lambswool. Something you can grab a hold of, run your hands (not fingers) through it. Rub, squeeze, and feel soft thick woolly hair. I've learned it's really about how we look at beauty, and what we have been made to perceive as beauty, subjectively.

I have gone through all the hair trips around. I've lost entire heads of hair, over and over again, with every new chemical made to straighten hair. Until finally one day, after losing yet another beautiful head of hair to a most infamous product, I decided "Enough!!!" I've got to learn to love the hair my Maker masterminded for me. Now don't get me wrong, there is nothing wrong with brand name perms and relaxers if you must, but don't you get tired of being dependent upon chemicals and hot irons because your hair is in that in-between growth stage, and you wouldn't be caught with the kink showing? When you travel you have to carry every hard and heavy hot metal iron you can lug. And what about your dependency on professional hair care specialists just to shampoo, condition, and style your hair? The costs! And if you are not in a Chocolate City like Detroit, a hair capital like Los Angeles, or any Black urban city anywhere in the world, what about finding a salon that has the professionals who are even familiar with the special needs of Black hair.

The styles with relaxers are pleasing, but temporary. Because of the constant adversity relaxed hair goes through as it grows out, however slowly it happens, it eventually seems to thin out and disappear, thereby never appearing to really grow at all. There's also something else to consider. The scalp, which is skin, absorbs those chemicals over the many years we use them. No matter how careful the relaxer is applied to "new growth only", the pores in the body absorbs those chemicals. You still feel the burning sensation on the scalp. You still smell the chemicals. I personally know people who had to stop receiving relaxer treatments because of health problems to the scalp and skin.

Eventually, as one get older, the skin becomes dryer and much more sensitive to harsh chemicals. It's to your advantage to have a strong, healthy scalp loaded with thick natural hair so you have some you can afford to lose with natural old age one day anyway.

So this book is an attempt to share the passion of learning to love my own natural, woolly, kinky, nappy hair with you my Sisters. We CAN grow our natural hair. It just takes a different appreciation, understanding, and attitude when approaching our natural hair and it's unique properties. We don't have to live with chemicals, and two separate textures of hair. We don't have to live with the terror of humidity "reverting" and revealing our true hair.

There's nothing wrong with locks. I find them beautiful, although they can be a bit confining for a woman whose taste includes hair variety. Sometimes you may choose a straight style, or an "ethnic" style, sometimes an upswept, or sculptured style. But two different textures of hair (as your perm grows out) is problematic if you want to maintain long, strong, healthy, thick hair. As an actress, I may supplement wigs, extensions, etc. if needed. I may need to go from "ethnic" to straight back to "ethnic" again, all in one week. But when I'm not working, I just want to be me, wearing my true hair texture, knowing I am still naturally beautiful and feeling good about myself without being dependent upon hair people, hair irons, hair money, or anything.

This book is dedicated to all of those Sisters with thick, coily, kinky, nappy, woolly hair who just want to be their natural beautiful selves. To every Sister who has heard the words kinky, nappy, peasy, or beady to describe their hair texture as if it was negative or unattractive. To all those Sisters who think they have "bad" hair or even ugly hair, because it takes a little more time to handle, or because it's not represented, or gloriously, commercially-celebrated, in mainstream America as "normal" hair. Anything worth having is worth taking more time to have. If one wants to maintain thick, long "virgin" hair, it takes attention, time, and care no matter what type of hair you may have naturally. If one doesn't have the time, energy, or understanding of our unique and different hair characteristics, then relaxers, wigs, and temporary hair is the ("convenient") answer. Those who wish to grow and maintain thick, kinky healthy hair, this book is written to you. And you probably are at a crossroads seeking hair change answers anyway, which is why you are reading this book.

So here's to letting the kinks fly!

CHAPTER 1

THE JOURNEY

"You never find yourself until you face the truth."

Pearl Baily

1918-1990

THE JOURNEY

I had not seen my own natural, unprocessed, unstraightened hair in more years than I can honestly remember. Perhaps more than half of my life. I came up when Black people were going through major significant hair changes resulting from serious social changes. "Black" was a vicious word to use to describe someone along with any reference to "nappy head", or "kinky hair". I experienced the radical social change from greasy hard-pressed and relaxed hair, to the so-called "Afro" or "Natural", back to new and improved relaxers, evolving to braids, weaves, extensions, beads, etc. The reason I say radical is because one must really understand what it meant at one time in this country to be a Black woman with natural unpressed hair ("nappy hair"). It was so significant an issue that women were fired from their jobs for wearing their hair in "Naturals". White people in general associated the hair with militancy and rebellion against "the Establishment". At this time in our history, no self-respecting or dignified Black woman would be caught dead with the kinks starting to grow back (the dreaded "new-growth"), or what I have come to phrase as "kink phobia".

Things are a lot different nowadays in terms of how we as Black people (and even society at large) look at our hair. But at the same time, some things seem to have reverted back to the old ways. Because hair processes and materials have improved, weaves and bonds are virtually undetectable - almost. Relaxers are not as harsh as they used to be although they still slowly eat away at the condition of your hair. Even pressing pomades have improved, along with thermal protectors, which accompany heat maintained styles. Between the improved weaving methods, improved relaxers, and undetectable extensions, it looks like straight silky hair naturally grows from a Black woman's head.

That is why I say some ways of thinking have returned upon us. I see some young girls who wouldn't be caught with the "kink" showing or growing underneath their relaxer. They really don't know, we've been through this already. But at the same time, some of these young girls are a little more "free" in their hair choices than we were. They are not necessarily slaves to straight hair. But for those of an older generation, natural African kinky hair is just unsettling to them. They are still reeling from the unsettling shock of the "Afro". To this set of Black people, *Dread*locks are *Dread*ful. This set of Black women prefer to see themselves with straight European looking hair, no matter what price has to be paid for it. We will blindly withstand harsh chemicals that seep into the bloodstream over the years; we will hot press it within an inch of its life; we will suffer from ear burns, forehead burns, neck burns *(ouch)*, just to have and maintain straight silky hair. We are terrified of humidity and water because it *will* revert back to its natural state. Or, we will just keep it weaved forever, until it pushes back revealing the "bush" underneath making it look like a helmet sitting on top of the head if it's not attended to right away. And because most Americans are such hair neurotics and will judge your entire existence upon your hair texture, most of us are hesitant to go with locks even if we desire them because of job restraints, parochial attitudes from family and friends, or comments that may sound critical or insulting, seldom complimentary. I think we've all experienced at some point during a hair transition involving locks, braids, or just our plain natural naps, some person looking at you with a twisted up curious look on their face before they say something insulting to your face about your hair.

But, believe it or not, we sisters are not unique in having society claim judgment on our hairstyle of choice either. In the 40's and 50's, when white chicks decided to cut their long straight hair short to "bobs" and "layers", there were those comments from their husbands and family. ("Christ! What have you done to your hair?!"). The style was a hit anyway in large part due to movies and magazines. White movie stars sported their hair in sexy short flips and bobs; the style was accepted, and popularized. Women who sported short sassy bobs were considered fast, hot and hip, maybe even loose. And if you compare the old Time and Life Magazines to the old Ebony Magazines, you can plainly see how much assimilation mattered to us as a people because we copied all of our white sister's hairstyles with attractive hot pressed versions of our own. Actually, since most of us had trouble growing our hair long (because the hot comb and curlers burned and broke our hair off constantly) the shorter bobs and layered cuts were welcomed by us. White chicks set the hairstyles of that time because we copied and assimilated, without questioning, at one time in this country.

We <u>are</u> unique, though, when it comes to the punishment and torture that Black women endure socially and emotionally because of our natural hair texture, not just style, but <u>texture</u>. No woman in the world has been insulted and fired from her job for wearing her own natural hair <u>texture</u>, except Black women in America. Our hair texture is treated as if there is something inherently wrong with it. It must be pressed to be finished or presentable.

I submit that our kinky hair texture is directly related to our sense of self-esteem, to social acceptance from Blacks <u>and</u> Whites, and our sexual pride about ourselves relating to men and what they find sexy and attractive. I know of men who wouldn't be caught with a woman in braids, and I know men who love them. Some men have gradually grown to accept braids and locks. The fact that it's so important to a man is where all of our problems stem. Some nappy headed men want nothing romantically to do with a nappy haired woman. Go figure. I have seen White men who have chosen Black women with the tightest kink, yet a Black man might reject a woman on that basis alone. Most of the brothers that I may have shared my bookwritings with expressed enthusiastically how much they prefer natural Black hair, and that they wanted to purchase a book for someone they loved.

Although Black hair isn't the complete political symbol it used to be, there are still negative and positive associations with regard to texture. We wore "naturals" and "afros" because we were an oppressed people discovering and redefining ourselves. Nowadays, most kids are just having fun, changing their hair at whim. It's more of an art than symbolism, which is how it should be. But to some of the conservative establishment, kinky hair still represents a symbol of something negative. Something not quite normal or comfortably ubiquitous. Even the roles in film and TV we tend to be offered to portray are those that don't necessarily lend themselves to sexual fantasy, thus a woman with locked hair may not be celebrated as alluring or sexy. Lauryn Hill's video where she is sporting a pressed style and a locked style simultaneously, is a wonderful example of our natural rich beauty, versatility, and sensuality. How interesting it is that we look alluring either way, which makes our hair unique sculptured works of art, really. Lauryn, thank you for that video.

I used to be one of those sisters who just knew I had "bad" hair. When I saw my cousin go from her pressed short hair to a "natural" (and she was a true pioneer having been one of the first at my high school to sport a "natural"), I was shocked. Then when I decided to bravely embrace the kink of my nature, by transforming my thick, neck-length pressed hair into an "afro", everyone around me was mildly shocked. Then, it began to grow on me as we took Black History classes, (which were just beginning to be put into schools), and we learned who we were and where we came from. We came to know and understand about our assimilation. At one time, it was like we were a sub-culture not even represented in magazines like TIME, LIFE, or NEWSWEEK, and since there was no "information age", a student was at the mercy of a school system which referred to us as "Negroes". Then Malcolm X began to preach praises of our kinky hair ancestry and refute notions that our hair was inferior or shameful in any way. A lot of Blacks shunned the straightening comb and sported "The Afro", with Pride. We were no longer ashamed of our woolly hair, but proud to be different. James Brown said it "loud". We were Black and we were Proud. Even <u>he</u> traded his beautifully coifed "process" in for a "natural". That's how important this entire movement of hair was. In order for him to sing the glory of what that song meant to us and our experience in America, it was important for the true Godfather of Soul to wear that "natural", and wear it he did.

Then we graduated to "cornrows", and people were repelled and appalled once again. That was going a little too far back to Africa. Black people were just starting to accept "naturals" among ourselves, but these flat braided cornrows parted so that the scalp showed had to go! (pickaninny! no!!!) I sported those cornrows, because by now I was archive and knee-deep into learning about our African-American History and social attitudes in this country. I wore those cornrows and heard all kinds of insults. Not from enlightened people though, which were few.

Then the "extensions" came to make your braids appear longer with secret added hair or beads, and that upset people too. "Is all that your real hair?", we were constantly demanded of by white women, as if long hair was their exclusive domain. Then the "extension" transformed into aesthetic works-of-art, and have progressed a long way since it's origin. Most Americans think they just came into vogue in the 90's, but that's the TV and film industry attempting to catch up to our reality.

So here we are in this day and age, still being antagonized because of our hair texture. A few years ago (late 90's), there were Black women being fired from their jobs at major airlines for wearing beautiful braids. Why? Even now certain anchor women or airline hostesses are expected to wear their hair straight, pressed, or relaxed. Braids or locks would be questioned, or unacceptable. So once again, the establishment is reminding us to repress who we are. To go through changes over our hair texture to fit their ideas of what is beautiful and socially acceptable. If our white sisters can wear long hairpieces, we ought to be allowed to wear long braid pieces.

What an unfair subliminal message this says about "natural" Black women. What seemingly innocuous discrimination Black women still endure, when things appear so free and progressive, as long as we conform.

So on my journey through this Black woman's hair, I'm learning again to deal with my own nappy, kinky, woolly, thick, curly, coily hair with Pride. I'm learning to love my hair, and actually <u>prefer</u> it in its non-straight existence. The information in this book is designed to communicate with those sisters who are desperate with chemicals and seeking truth and change; therefore, the references herein regarding "our hair" is in the language of those with relaxed hair, not the language of those who have already made the transition, but to those seriously considering a change and are a bit afraid.

To those sisters who have already reached the enlightenment of natural or locked hair, I say Congratulations. You are truly free. Chemical free. Perhaps this book will provide entertaining confirmation of what you have already discovered and experienced.

By the way, from this reading point on, we will write "dreadlocks" as "dredlocks", or just plain "locks". We will no longer even subliminally think of our natural hair in any terms of dread or negativity.

I LOVE BRAIDS

I have worn my braids at this writing for about four years now allowing my hair a much needed rest so it could thicken and grow, returning to its' natural state. It has been wonderful to rediscover the texture of my hair and realize how truly soft it is. I hadn't seen my own hair in so long that I assumed my hair to be hard and ugly when it's actually soft and pleasing to the touch.

I began wearing braids after a most distressing experience with the infamous RIO Hair Relaxer System. A most destructive hair relaxer which was advertised on national television to Black women who were desperately looking for something to relax their hair without harsh chemicals, and the high price dependency of salon visits. The actors even ate the product on TV to prove that there were no harsh chemicals in it. The culprit owners got rich, and disappeared. There was a huge class action lawsuit, and broken hair, and broken self-esteem abounded everywhere.

After years of looking for that magic hair "convenience", that magic product that would finally alter or change the texture of my hair without harsh chemicals, I was willing to try anything. That's always where the problem starts: wanting to change the texture of our hair. Wanting it somehow silky straight. I was sucked into a fraudulent advertisement that ruined my hair so bad that I finally decided I had to find another way. And they knew just how to market it to us. Hair that moved! Hair soft and bouncy! Easy to maintain! You can do it yourself. Mild, Natural, and Inexpensive!

This product was so vicious that it undermined us by eating away our hair slowly, so that the real damage might not show up until two or three shampoos later. It did something strange to the color of my natural light ash brown hair making it some indiscernible dark and strange color. I could sort of live with that, but then it became unmanageable, dry, and wiry. It snapped off constantly in the comb. It wouldn't hold a style. I was losing it uncontrollably every day, and what was left was like straw. It seemed nothing would arrest the continuing damage. Those who continued with touch-up applications, lost ALL of their hair.

I was too ashamed to call my beloved hair dresser again with this self-inflicted damage, so I sucked up the embarrassment, went to the store, purchased a good cholesterol super-detangling conditioner for extremely damaged hair, called my local braider, and began making regular visits over a period of almost four years.

I have a thick beautiful head of natural "virgin" hair now.

So that I could reacquaint myself with my own hair, I would take my hair down in tiny stages instead of all at once. I would wear bangs in front that I lightly blow-dried and hot curled, and the rest braided long down my back. That way I had a chance to play with my new hair texture (which had become foreign to me). I wasn't overwhelmed all at once with a head full of thick long bushy hair and not a clue of what to do with it.

The greatest thing about braids is the ease of daily maintenance. You are relieved of comb-carrying, and yet you always look nicely groomed, even after leaving a hot sweaty gym, or lovemaking. (And as far as I'm concerned that's a big plus. My husband thinks so too). Another little secret treat worth mentioning is the slight temporary "face-lift" you get when you pin or tie the braids up off of your face. Scrunchies and hairpins are real helpful for those styles.

The bottom line is that braids free me up from always fussing with my hair in between shampoos. I found that when I traveled, I always had more time to devote to early rising, sightseeing, and late night parties. I had more time to be on-the-go. When traveling to places like Europe or the Bahama Islands, it is of special importance not to have hair traumas. The electrical outlets in other countries are not always compatible with a lot of those "special tools" we carry when maintaining relaxed or pressed hairstyles. And if you like to swim (as I do), braids are total common sense when overseas.

BRAIDERS

I was very fortunate to know not only a good braider at the time of my last "emergency", but an outstanding one. I've had many sisters braid my hair throughout the years. Some were just friends doing me a favor, so it may take all night and a bottle of wine and cheese to get through most of my head. Some used me as practice, but never charged me, and went on to become great braiders with their own flourishing businesses. But at the time and in the city of my last emergency, I was blessed to know someone who had become a really skilled braid-artist. Because of her, whenever I look for a braider, there are certain traits and principles that are a must.

First and foremost, she (or he) must be *fast.* That's my absolute first priority. Time is of vital importance these days. Many sisters don't consider braids because of that one factor. It takes serious time. This sister I knew was phenomenal, and she was proud of it. We both knew of salons that would charge top dollar, put two people on one head, and still take longer than it would take her to finish.

I liked to wear long single braids all over my head long enough for me to sit on. What fun that is. Sometimes I would get them in multi-colors to match the highlights in my hair. That's a demanding style that would take an amateur days to complete ("Girl, come back tomorrow..."). My braider was a serious professional. Even though she was a friend of mine, she was all business. I really liked that. I knew of a few skilled braiders, but not necessarily superfast ones. I sported a thick head full of waist-length multi-colored braids in four hours! That's comparable to the time it takes to go to a salon, wait your turn, get your hair done, and hope it doesn't rain next week. It's a long day at the beauty parlor, if you have a fast braider, not one who gets up every few minutes to do something, eat something, etc. Sometimes she would actually braid two people in one day! She was astonishingly fast. I was always scheduled early in the morning. She would start at 8 a.m., and I'm leaving her house by noon with a gorgeous hairstyle that will last for weeks or months. I can go swimming, get caught in the rain, engage in the sweatiest "activities", and still look my best, and not fuss with my hair afterward. Not to mention that my hair itself is resting, growing, and becoming healthy again. There's no daily tug, fuss, and stress on the hair. No costly burn accidents from trying to touch it up yourself.

Now don't misunderstand. There is a type of maintenance for braids. They must be groomed, oiled, and conditioned, not allowed to just become dry ratty hair, especially if there is any chemical work done to your own hair. Synthetic braids tend to really hold up over time. You can shampoo them and spread conditioner on them. Afterward use lots of absorbent towels to wrap around the braids like sponges. If it's hot outside, you can go out and dry naturally which is always best. If you are in cold weather, you can blow-dry the braids and scalp, or sit under a traditional hood dryer.

Make sure you use an emollient leave-in conditioner after your rinse-out. I love adding a few drops of essential oils to my favorite leave-in for a sensuous aroma. I'll add a drop of vanilla, clove, or perhaps sandalwood. In the summer I'll even play around lightly with jasmine or rose for a more sweet flowery scent in the hair. Light pomades are sufficient for relaxed hair but I find "natural" hair is constantly absorbing moisture, so heavier emollients are advisable when it comes to keeping your braids conditioned. You should experiment until you find the right hairdressing conditioner for you. The book *"Good Hair...For Colored Girls Who've Considered Weaves When the Chemicals Became To Ruff"*, by Lonnice Brittenum Bonner is an excellent supplemental reference for enlightenment on handling and conditioning natural hair. Her research is quite thorough and invaluably informative. As a matter of fact, her book was extremely inspiring and helpful for me personally. I'd lost long entire heads of hair several times in my life. I've had to crop it extremely short many times as a result of serious hair damage. Her entertaining and candid book gave me the courage to begin a new hair life.

The second most important requirement for a braider is quality and skill. Is she good? Does she understand what you want and can she deliver to your happy satisfaction, because once it's braided, it's braided. Does she tug and pull unnecessarily hard at your hair while braiding? My braider had the hands of a masseuse, and the high quality skill of her trade. I received many compliments (even from anti-braid people sometimes surprisingly). Her skilled perfection allowed me to wear them for long lengths of time (up to six months once!). Eventually I would cut them into different lengths, creating a totally new style before I took the braids out. I might hot-water curl them, or hot water dip them straight. Once dry, I would unravel them on the bottom allowing the tight kinky waves to flow which actually sort of looked like the stuff growing from my scalp, which is why I strongly recommend synthetic hair as your own natural fuzziness starts to show itself. It actually sort of matches that hair better than the very expensive human hair because it tends to have a matching kink illusion of all one texture.

As I experimented with the synthetic vs. human hair, I noticed that the synthetic always received compliments. White people who were strangers would approach me with, "Is that all your hair?" (as if they had a right to know). They would break all rules of social politeness and demand, perhaps even on a crowded elevator, "Is that all your hair?" And if it only happened once, it would not be worth mentioning, but it happened constantly, no matter what city I was in. "Is that all your hair?", only from white folks. The fact that it made them so curious that they just had to ask no matter how inappropriate or rude, let me know how nice the work must be that my braider did. So, yes, quality is my second most important priority.

My third priority is cost. Even though I believe in paying for what you get, I don't wish to be overcharged, but when it comes to the crowning glory, I'm not necessarily frugal either. I wouldn't want to abuse a fast, reliable braider's time, effort, and skill by being cheap. I'd like to think I always treated my braider with the utmost respect by generously tipping her as well as I could afford to do. Haggling over price sells the entire session short. Being fair and generous, (and not asking for credit, please) always guaranteed respect for my appointments, and squeeze-ins whenever I called at the last minute (because of the nature of my unpredictable work). After all, a good braider is in demand and will always have a schedule to be reckoned with. Getting on her schedule should always be made a priority if you are serious about a growing program for your hair. Occasionally, I would make my next appointment in advance even if it was three months away. Advance appointments also have another advantage in that it allows yourself a time table for not only taking down your hair, but shampooing, conditioning, and even giving a little clip on the ends. Stretching it out a little with the blow dryer kept down the kinks, made her job fast, and my costs for her time fair.

BRAID REMARKS & COMMENTS

I knew a young lady of Persian ethnicity at my music classes. She was a receptionist who genuinely admired my lovely braids every time she saw me. Finally, one day she asked me about having her own shoulder-length straight hair braided - like mine! Imitation is the most sincere form of flattery, and I was happy to send my fantastic braider another customer (not that she needed it).

My music class happened to be in a white part of town, and my braider was in “the Hood”. After the receptionist made the appointment with my braider, she told me her boyfriend forbade her from getting “those pickaninny things” in her hair. He wouldn’t be seen with a pickaninny and that the braids would damage her hair anyway. He informed her that the Black part of Los Angeles was dangerous and that the men would attack her. No, this wasn’t 1960 or even the 1930’s, but 1997!! Gorgeous young sisters are sporting braids in their music videos, and TV shows, and this is the sentiment of an uninformed young man toward braids and Black women in 1997! Well, it’s an awful sentiment anytime, but especially at a time when we are being lulled into thinking everything is equal, sophisticated, and relaxed.

Anyway, the receptionist told me what her boyfriend said, and I told her I would not send her somewhere dangerous. I would not go somewhere dangerous, myself. And, that I knew her boyfriend had to be white. He was. She insisted on having her hair braided though, so, accompanied by her brothers and uncles, she went to "the Hood". My braider's dexterity was so fascinating to watch, it amazed them; and her hair was so lovely, in such a short time, that they were humbled and awed at the work (not to mention her immaculate and pristine place of business). She insisted on wanting her braids "as long as Ella's!". My braider took her to the store to match her own lovely straight hair with an exact human hair match. The girl was whistled at and complimented so, even her narrow minded boyfriend chilled out, and she became a regular customer.

But my point is that compliments are great. We all like them, but enduring verbal opinions laced with insult, and ignorant or rude comments is the stuff that the mettle of a Black woman is made from, especially when it comes to our kinks and braids. And they come from everywhere, sometimes where you least expect - family, friends, co-workers, bosses, lovers, even strangers. The anti-braid/anti-Black woman sentiment is exhausting, discriminating, and parochial. It can actually make people say aggressive, hurtful, and ignorant things that you just have to be strong enough to ignore, overcome, or perhaps show enduring patience, by considering the source of the remark.

I could go on and on in a book alone dedicated to the nice and not so nice comments I've heard over the years regarding my braids and naps, but there are other things I want to cover in this book, so I'll just a recall a few. For those of you reading this book and already are braidwearers (or hairlocked sisters) some of these comments will probably be entertainingly familiar:

"Braids break your hair off." No, braids grow your hair out. Anything breaks and damages your hair if not maintained properly. If you don't condition a perm, you will dry and break your hair. If you don't condition color-treated hair or highlights, your hair will disappear. If you don't condition your braids, yes, they may break and damage your hair. If you don't use patience taking them out, yes, you will break your hair off, or snatch your hair out. If you dye, tint, or lighten your hair and immediately braid it up afterward, yes, you will damage and break it. You should wait at least six weeks before you re-braid after coloring, always deep conditioning the hair until then.

Now, I am not a hair professional by any means. I am not licensed, but I do have a thick head of hair as a result of constantly wearing braids for three to four years. It's thicker and longer than it has been all of my life. A salon didn't do it. *I did it.* And you can too. If you can quietly stand up to all the uncalled for comments and remarks, knowing in a few years some of those same people will be jealous to see all of that thick lush hair you are going to end up with, believe me, it will be worth it.

"That's your hair and everyone else's isn't it?" Nice loud comment for the entire office to hear. She's just looking for a way to put you down. She doesn't want any man to possibly think that all of that hair is really yours.

"If I see one more black and gold braid... I just can't take it." This comment is from someone who gave up on her hair and cut it all off until almost bald. Once again, consider the source.

"It takes too long.... I can't sit that long." That's legitimate. But even if it takes all day, it's one long day that's worth it for beauty, comfort, and long-term convenience.

"It's so expensive". Those same people will spend $200 at a salon for "the works" that will last until a good work-out session at the gym, yet your $150 braid extension style lasts two, three, maybe even five months. Go figure. And of course there are styles much less expensive than long, single braid extensions.

"How do you guys get those <u>things</u> in your hair?" Intended to be complimentary but somehow always sounds condescending and insulting. Besides, I am not a "guy".

"She was wearing dreadlocks..." No, she was wearing *braids*. Referring to *braids* as "dreadlocks" always grates a nerve.

Some fellow whites are actually sensitive and cultivated enough about our hair culture to not offend. So instead of, "Is all that your hair?", they'll say perhaps, "I like your hair", or "I love your new hairstyle", not "I like your *extensions*". You know, white movie starlets have worn hair pieces and hair extending secrets for decades, especially in the movies. But then again the "faux" or false hair available to them was made to perfectly match their true hair texture, strand per strand. Not always the same case with us. Silky hair does not generally grow from a kinky-haired woman's scalp. It's another *feel* altogether. Not better or worse, it just has to be appreciated differently. Touched and handled differently. We all have some variety of kink or curl at the roots. Some have wavy kinky curl, some have fuzzy kinky curl - all types, which is why we can get away with wearing so many different grades of wigs, even silky hair, if we choose.

And, of course, the sophisticated and enlightened people complimented me constantly in a classy way. I recall an Englishman once say to me at an airport, "However long that took, it certainly was worth it. Your hair is quite lovely".

The comments go on and on, but you get the picture. If you're lucky enough to find a great braider, go ahead and braid it until it grows to the long, thick, healthy length you desire, and ignore the strange comments.

LONG BRAIDS vs. SHORT BRAIDS

You can get long braids or short braids. Short braids are of course quicker and cheaper, especially if using synthetic hair. You can even get multi-colored braids, auburn, blonde, gray, even blue! But the length usually determines time, money, and believe it or not, attention.

I was chatting with a fellow actress friend of mine, and we were so tickled comparing our notes at how differently men treat you when you wear long hair braids compared to short braids. We both cracked up laughing at how men broke their necks to open a door for you if your braids were down to your butt. They smile, take notice, flirt, say "Hi!" to you, and are just nicer in general when we wear long braids.

Conclusion: Men love long hair. Lots of hair. Most of them. No matter what they say, watch how they behave. Men like thick, long hair on women. Nowadays, they don't even seem to care if it's store bought or not, just long. As a matter of fact, people in general seem amazingly nicer to me with long braids or hair. Go figure America. Have you ever read the book or saw the old movie, *"Black Like Me"*, where the main white character actually changes his appearance to that of a "Negro" (with injections), so he could experience just how poorly "the colored" were treated in society? It astounded him. Be a Black woman in America and try changing your hair with a purpose from braids, to nappy afro, and then wear long straight hair, and compare the differences in how you are perceived and treated. It's a deep experience.

TAKING YOUR BRAIDS OUT

Think of your hair as a tangle of very fine 14k gold chains, and you <u>must</u> unravel them. **Patience** is the key word here. If you snatch them out in a hurry, the hair will break and snap. That's common sense that a lot of women don't practice. And, yes, you <u>can</u> unlock locked hair if you leave the braids in too long. Never past six months though if you don't want real trouble. Once the dredlocks are really long, there is no turning back without cutting, but I have actually unlocked hair that was over one inch in length. ***Patience.*** Hair will begin to naturally lock after four to five weeks in braids anyway, but the key to unlocking the hair is **patience** and **intense conditioners**.

I remember this neurotic actress I worked with once who happened to have mixed children. She was one of those who thought she was an expert on Black people since she was married to a Black man, and had absolutely no Black female friends. She was looking at my braids one day, and of course the negativity couldn't contain itself, and she had to inform me how bad the braids were for her daughter's hair, and for Black women in general. Her daughter who evidently did not inherit her mother's straight silky hair, but some of her daddy's "kink". Well, her daughter wanted braids for the summer, against her mother's will, and when she took them out there were "knots" all over her head, and her mother felt she had to cut off her entire head of hair and start over (as punishment). She wasn't interested in finding out what she didn't know because she was so highly opinionated on Black hair, Black people, Black anything, that she certainly didn't need a Black <u>woman</u> to tell her anything about her Black daughter's nappy hair. Her attitude and conversation was so anti-braid (laced with a little "kink-phobia" and a lot of "kink-denial" thrown in), that I just kept quiet and kept the "secret" to myself as she prattled on and on, but I wanted to tell her how unnecessary it was to cut off all of that new growth. I also wanted her to know that if we as Black women are still trying to figure out the unique kink-and-curl properties and characteristics of our own natural hair, what makes her such an authority? She could have saved all of her daughter's kinky curly hair with time, patience, and appreciation, meaning not dealing with kinky hair as if it's supposed to be straight. Go with the hair, not against it.

Black African hair is supposed to be super curly or tight curly. Deal with it that way as you take it down. The kinkier it is, the dryer it can be, so coat each braid with your choice of oil, pomade, or African Nut Shea butter (which I highly recommend), along with a conditioner like Lustrasilk's super-detangling creme conditioner (in the green jar). It's a must for unintentionally locked hair. Once it softens, begin to gently pull apart each strand of hair. Just like a knot of fine gold chains. Yes, it takes a lot of time and patience the longer you have worn it into its' locked state. I've done this many, many times throughout the past three to four years that I've worn braids to grow my hair out, affording me the opportunity to become very intimate with the touch, feel, and natural charactistics of my kinks; not trying to eradicate them, but cherish them. I have a thick head of hair to show for it. No hair loss.

Nowadays, there are a lot more products available to sisters which are actually labeled to "remove knots and braids", because we are rediscovering our hair roots all the time, it seems. After you've gently pulled that single lock of hair loose, you will need to comb it out immediately. Do this with each braid. Hair will come out in the comb, but it's the normal daily hair loss that has been tied up in the braid and not removed, so don't panic! That's usually what happens when a severe haircut is the result of wearing braids a few weeks too long.

Do each locked braid like that one at a time. Every couple of braids, comb out all the exposed hair, clip or twist it out of the way, and proceed to the next braid. When you get an entire section of hair released and combed out, twist it up out of the way. Try to have four or six large sections of hair, and wash it that way, combing it out with a very wide tooth comb, or good quality Afro Pik, or rake. Wash, condition, and comb each large section separately. Take your time if you want to save your hair. Never take all of your braids out at once without having combed the tiny sections of hair first. You will get tangled and frustrated trying to manage it all. You'll be tempted to cut and relax for sure. You should never just shampoo your natural hair without a softening and loose comb-out first, anyway. You can do that with natural straight hair, but not with thick Black virgin hair.

I remember one time my husband and I were on location in Canada. I unbraided my braids. It hadn't reached the locked stage yet; I had worn them for only a conservative two weeks. It was pretty easy to take down. I slipped into the shower, without combing it out first. I shampooed, conditioned, and attempted to comb it out. I couldn't! I had approached my hair as if it were straight and silky. After all, I still had a perm. I thought the loose hair would just rinse right out. I thought the comb would just glide through the hair. It was a jungle mess. I panicked! No, I freaked!! I'm way up in

Canada somewhere, where even if they have a Black hair corner in the back of the store on the bottom shelf somewhere, it's not going to have the specialized products *I* desperately needed at the time. Do you remember that funny commercial where the lady had tried some new product on her hair and she was in the bathroom crying loud Lucille Ball-type "boo hoos", and her husband was sitting on the bed, genuinely concerned, saying, "Honey, it's not that bad", and she just cried louder? Well, that was me. Wet, frazzled, and mildly hysterical as my genuinely concerned husband heroically ran out into the dark white wilds of Canada to harpoon me a super detangling intensive conditioner - somewhere. What a man. He found something, and it took me all night to untangle my hair, and eventually get the comb through it. I didn't want to lose my hair, and that's how I discovered the patience of untangling locked and overly tangled hair - *strand by patient strand.*

New growth on relaxed hair <u>must</u> be reckoned with gently so it doesn't break. Always comb it out before you shampoo and soften it before you comb. Use a small fine tooth comb as you pick loose each small single braid. Then switch to an extra wide tooth comb or Afro Pik to comb the large sections of hair. Comb the ends of the hair first, moving up toward the scalp. With relaxed hair, you shampoo and comb it out afterward. I find with natural kinky hair, it's better handled to comb <u>as</u> I shampoo so that I'm not overwhelmed with too many kinks at once. Remember, we are changing our entire idea of how to handle our hair. Straight hair can be combed right from the scalp, and that was the mistake I made in Canada by attempting to comb it out all at once from the scalp.

Never attempt to comb out dry, kinky hair. It will break. Why would you even want to comb out a dry kink from the scalp anyway? Why? Don't you know it's going to hurt? Why would you attempt to scrape an Ace comb through a head full of dry kinks and naps? Because that's how we are programmed to handle hair, that's why. Straight hair. That Ace comb is designed for hair that lays flat and straight, not a head full of dry springy kinks. There's one entertaining moment in Ms. Bonner's book were she described the little girl running away from the Ace comb that I know will sound familiar to a lot of sisters. It is only because of our straight hair foundation that we would even attempt to comb a head full of dry springy kinks with a comb made for straight flat hair. Another friend of mine shared with me stories of her little girl's short tight kinky hair breaking up many combs in the house. It's not her fault that our society's preference for hairstyle is straight hair care. Natural kinks are easier to handle with an oil moisturizer or spray detangler first. Kinks and tangles are easier to handle when gently pulled apart by the fingers, (not snatching a comb through it from the scalp). Natural kinks are also easier to handle in sections, opposed to the entire head at once.

Everything doesn't always work for everyone's hair type, but what I hope to do here is share kinky hair "tips" for dealing specifically with kinky virgin hair, hoping to stimulate your own creative juices when it comes to styling this type of natural hair. Moisturized and conditioned "virgin" hair is stronger than processed hair. I could never tug and pull on my relaxed hair without snapping a few strands off, but kinky hair <u>can</u> break combs. Virgin hair has strong tensile strength. Our natural hair is strong. It will grow long and not break, if treated correctly. If it's allowed to dry out, it breaks. If combed as if it were straight in nature, it breaks. Treat it according to its own unique curly properties and it grows strong. If your natural hair is very thick, bushy, and kinky, (the break-an-Ace-comb kind of kink), then leave that comb alone! Style with your hands. You really don't have to resort to chemicals. By leaving the entire "daily comb and brush" concept alone, you will create new, naturally pleasing hairstyles.

BRAID RITUALS

One more word on braids to share with you is the sheer ritual of it. They create a bond between Black women. If you are as fortunate as I was to have your own *personal* braider, you really have an advantage for a grow-braid program. You may have to try a few braiders before you find a reliable professional just right for you, but when you do find her, stick with her, and take care of her. By that I mean tip her generously. Be on time for appointments. Wash and condition your hair before your appointment. Personally, I would even blow-dry and stretch my hair out before I went to make her job effortless. I did not want to spend more time than necessary. The only time we stopped was for bathroom breaks, tea, and a little stretch of the legs.

If you are really fortunate, you will find someone you like chatting with as well, bonding the sisterhood of our Black hair experience. Because our kinks are so misunderstood and so very personal to us, it helps to be able to chat candidly about our kinky hair, bonding Black women in the similar way our music and dance does. It bonds us because of our common social experience in America. It bonds us because of society's kink-phobia. I'm always amazed by the hypocrisy of a society who in 1920 gave all American women the right to vote, but those of kinky haired ancestry were not included in the heart of that document. African American women would not see its inclusion until the Civil Rights struggles of the 60's.

So the kink, the dredlock, the knotty braids are uniquely our own experience in America. When sisters are braiding hair, it's a wonderful (maybe even unspoken) bond that I take delight in. It's our secret sister club.

KNOTS

If the braids are only four or five weeks in, when you remove them you will probably have knots instead of real locks. Coat the knot at the scalp with oils, and creme conditioner. Rub the knot between your fingers allowing the knot to absorb the emollient oils. It will soften and loosen. Gently hold the knot with your left hand, and with the right index finger and thumb, loosen and pull the hair free out of the knot. If you've coated it generously, it will slide backwards out of the knot (towards the scalp). Do this a few strands at a time. Be sure to pin or clip the other braids or loose hair completely out of the way as you release your lubricated knots. You will get tangled and frustrated if the other hair gets in your way. Also, you may lose your knot-spot when you take your arms down for a rest, so it's easier to find that knot at the back of your head if you clip the other hair out of the way.

You will end up with a knot of loose hair in your left hand to discard. These are the strands of hair that naturally loosened during the time it's been braided and tied up. It's a normal loss or shed of hair. The hair on your head has grown longer. You must be patient, so just plan on evenings of looking at TV with a jar of shea butter and your favorite super-detangling conditioner. Keep telling yourself, "I want long, thick hair", and you will find the patience to unravel the new growth, strand by strand, if you have to.

As Shakespeare wrote, "Vanity, thy name is woman".

LOCKS (Unintentional)

Six months of braids will definitely give you locks. If you desire dredlocks, then braids into dredlocks is an easy yet sexy and attractive way to transform. Personally, I'm not fond of the short-short dreds on myself. I like them on men. Some sisters look great and very sexy because they truly have the face and headshape for the look. But for those sisters who truly feel they need hair of some sort framing their face, you can just let your own hair begin to lock naturally underneath synthetic braids.

The book, *Everything You Need To Know About Hairlocking"*, by Nekhena Evans, is a serious read for anyone seriously considering permanently locking their hair. Her insight and research is extremely enlightening even if you are only considering the big step of just going natural, not necessarily locking. It inspired me. I strongly recommend reading it.

On the other hand, if you are going through a hair grow-braid program, and your hair is four to six months in braids, you have the beginning of locks. Super-detangling creme is absolutely necessary. Use the one for damaged hair (although we have established that your hair is not damaged. It is only locked). Apply it generously all over the lock, and with a fine tooth comb or the end of a hair pin, gently pick the hair apart from the bottom up. Once again, some of the strands will come out and that is normal. Those strands that are strongly rooted in your scalp will remain unless you lose patience and start tugging and snatching. Take your time generously oiling and creaming the hair as you go. You may have to reapply the creme and oil several times because your thirsty virgin hair will constantly absorb the moisture as you detangle it. It's okay to really coat it on because you're going to shampoo that section anyway.

Ideally, you should take the braids down before the hair starts locking, but sometimes that's not the case. There were times when I've been on the road with a play and my hair was in braids resting while I wore wigs for my stage role. Under a demanding theater schedule there is absolutely no time to fool around with your hair. Whenever I would return home, my hair would have small dredlocks. Since I chose not to lock it right now, I used the method I just described discovering this method as I went. The first time I had locks or "knots", I panicked. And since all of the traditional and conservative beauticians want to admonish and discourage you from locking or "damaging" your hair in the first place, I didn't want to deal with a scolding. After reading *"Everything You Need To Know About Hairlocking"* and *"Good Hair"*, I was inspired, and acquired a totally different attitude and understanding about my hair.

The first thing was to calm down, and stay in control of my natural hair. Not be afraid of it. I refused to cut it. I grabbed large dollops of creme conditioner and smothered my hair and scalp. I used olive oil as well. My hair soaked up the moisture. It became soft and manageable. I spent several hours a day gently pulling apart a few braids each day. Then, I would wash and comb just the exposed section, not the entire head necessarily.

I discovered plenty of attractive ways to twist or pin the exposed unbraided hair each day. The fact that your hair is part braided and part loose need not be an anxious point of concern. It gives you the opportunity to ease into re-discovering your own hair texture. By experimenting with gels, pomades, creme butters and oils in small twists and twirls, you will begin to stimulate ideas for styling. You can even blow-dry the small amount of exposed hair, or you can hot curl press it out of habit, but this is the most opportune time to introduce yourself to twisting it. It won't be time consuming, because it's only a small amount of exposed hair you are experimenting with. The rest is still braided. I'll go more into detail about styling that exposed hair later in Chapter 3 - "MAINTAINING NATURAL HAIR.

HAND GROOMING

As you begin to release your hair from the braids and more of your own natural hair is exposed, use that opportunity to begin to experiment with your own hair texture. If the perm is still present, be extra careful with the hair, because it will continue to be weak. Those relaxed and porous ends can get tangly in an unnatural way. Gently pull them apart with your fingers, not the comb. Eventually they have to go, revealing your true hair texture.

A good rich pomade or hairdressing is a must when you are wearing part braids and part loose hair. Your dry hair will absorb it. Smear generous amounts of oils and conditioners on your hands, and knead the hair grabbing large amounts of hair and braids at a time, rubbing your hands - not fingers - on the hair, not through the hair, as if it was straight. As it softens, gently pull it apart styling the hair around your crown. Your hair will be conditioned by soaking up the oils and moisture. I highly recommend African Nut Shea butter when handling dry hair. The African kinky hair seems to love it. (The ashy skin loves it too!)

KINK PHOBIA

"Kink". We can barely acknowledge the word. "Kinks". We can barely say it. Kinky hair. Why does that word scare us so? Repel us so? Offend us so? Straight hair is fine. Curly hair may be fine. But the sound of the phrase "kinky hair" sends us into fits of denial, filled with phobia. (Phobia is taken from the Greek work "phobus" - to fear or dread).

What's amazing to me now is how society has attempted to copy us. The white actress, Bo Derek, wore braids in the movie "10", at a time when Black women were being fired from their professional jobs for even wearing braids. Some of the "hippies" curled and teased their hair up tight to a curly nappy frizz during the militant radical unrest of the 60's and early 70's.

Do you remember the hair neurosis of most white Americans when The Beatles (with absolutely straight hair) appeared with their hair long? Not curled, mock-kinked, or frizzy, just long and straight. It was considered such an anti-establishment offense to some that certain white men wanted to fight and brawl over it. So you can just imagine the fits they had over *our* hair.

But the mid 70's actually saw commercialization of our new found hair identity. I was at first appalled when I saw "Afro" wigs in the stores commercializing our new found hair pride. At the end of the decade, it seemed they really went too far with the blue, green, and pink Afro wigs. Another decade later, you actually have braided and dredlocked wigs, for your convenience. And while our hair attitudes have somewhat simmered, and the wigs don't have the same stigma they used to have - a wig is still a wig. As a matter of fact, it seems as if Black women and wigs, weaves, and false hair have become a unique part of our culture. If you don't have time to coif your hair before an engagement, sometimes a wig is a great convenience. But what about just being afraid to be you? Afraid to let your true kinky hair show you as a sexy vibrant woman. I know Black women right now who have no idea what their own kinky virgin hair looks like. I was one of them. They've only been acquainted with the fuzz just starting to reveal itself before they are relaxing it again. Some do it every three weeks! Some do it right on time every month. They become slaves to the relaxer. One gentleman shared with me that he was glad I was writing this book, because his wife seemed to touch up her relaxer every week. He secretly wanted her to go with her natural hair, but she was afraid to give it a try.

I wore a relaxer many years. I was lucky to have fast growing thick hair, because I destroyed it many times. When you wear a relaxer, you can't help but suffer from kink phobia. Two different textures of hair lends itself to breakage and loss of hair texture control.

At first it gives fresh-relaxed hair a lot of beauty and straight lovely sleekness. After it grows out a week or two, it actually looks fuller and bouncier with a lot of body ("hair that moves!"). Then after another few weeks, it starts needing things like treatments. Then, if you don't re-relax it (or touch it up), you have the start of real problems. If you *tint and relax* it, without professional care, eventually that short cute haircut is waiting for you.

So if the 60's and 70's saw a lot of us with kinky cotton-soft afros and natural hair, why did we re-embrace the relaxers again in the 80's? (Or the really dreadful Jheri "scary" curls?) Many reasons I think. Many excuses too.

Politically, the current administration of the times brought a sort of anti-Black sentiment into the nation's capital, in my opinion. Conservatism was really a code name for racism. Straight hair became associated with being conservative. Afro anything was not really in style anymore. As a matter of fact, there was a sort of backlash against "Blackness". Many of us decided our "naturals" were limited to one type of hairstyle. Relaxers had improved, but the new no-lye relaxers still contained *chemicals* of some sort that eventually eat at the condition of your hair.

Let's understand - to permanently straighten Black hair bone straight, you must use a chemical. There is no herb that will do this permanently. By permanent, I mean after it is shampooed with water. It will not just fall bone straight without chemical help and heat. That is why we call relaxers "perms" because they are permanent. They permanently take curl out of our hair. "Perms" for Caucasian straight hair is to put body or curl *into* their hair because it will fall straight and limp after wetting it. So a "perm" for them, and a "perm" for us, has two different meanings.

The 80's saw many hair changes. Some grass root sisters never went back to straight hair. They began locking their hair slowly during this decade, and some were locked out of corporate employment as well. Some of us, (especially those of us in the conservative work force), felt we needed convenience, variety, and once again - conformity. You just were not going to be hired with dredlocks or natural bushy hair in certain professional jobs. Our society as we knew it was starting to speed up. Time and energy became increasingly important, so "To heck with this stuff, I'm relaxing it."

At that time I didn't quite understand like I do now, that it was only "difficult" because I was always only trying to style it into straight hair styles everyday. It's not so difficult if I choose to wear my natural hair in its' natural state emphasizing kinks, curls, and coils.

But Kink Phobia was with a lot of us and actually found it's way into the 90's. I'm not too sure I would have been casted on TV on *"Roc"* in 1991 wearing thick bushy hair or dredlocks. When the late great Rosalind Cash was cast to play my mother, I was pleasantly surprised and delighted. All of my sister friends in Detroit and Chicago just loved her locks. Here's a grass root sister who opted to be herself an entire decade before it was popular and accepted.

Before she passed away, she won a contract on General Hospital where we immensely enjoyed watching her in all of her hairlocked beauty. You could tell she had schooled the hair people on the set on handling and pinning her hair into glorious upsweeps. I often wondered if it was the first time any of them had actually put their hands upon dredlocks and kinky hair. They let her use her own natural style, and she was glorious on the show.

Nowadays, thanks to people like Rosalind Cash or Whoopi Goldberg, there is a bit of relaxation over braids, locks, and kinks, but not nearly enough. I would love to see them enhanced in our world of beauty. Have you ever seen a glamour hair or perfume ad, with a beautiful sister in a sexy gown with long, glorious braids or locks, or thick long kinks and naps? I would love to see a luscious woman of color and kinks getting "the urge", as a group of sexy men surround her in her hair glory on a network TV commercial. It seems the only place our visual hair beauty might be celebrated is in music videos. If a sister is in long luscious hairlocks, she may not necessarily land a position as a First Class flight attendant, although some attitudes are slowly changing. What has become disturbing is that braids and dredlocks tend to be associated with blue collar jobs. She just might get a job as clean-up personnel, but not a hostess. Black women with blue collar jobs, where they may not be visible to the public are okay, other professionals have to risk perhaps being fired, or not being hired in the first place.

Here's an interesting anecdote for you. It's the year 2000 while I'm feverishly writing this book, and just a few minutes ago on TV, there was an interesting news item on Channel 7. There's a high school somewhere here in Los Angeles, where students have been expelled for wearing their hair in large "afros". The authority figure who happened to be white was interviewed, and said that their rules were "no-braids, no outrageous hairstyles". (That's pretty subjective; outrageous to who?). The students' response was that the hairstyle is their proud heritage.

Now it is obvious that this rule is based on standards of Kink Phobia, but what's "outrageous" is that in December 2000, Black people are still antagonized about our hair.

So, at times, it seems to me we've come all the way from Black hair discrimination, back to Black hair discrimination, and straight hair assimilation back to straight hair assimilation. A few contemporary music artists have brought natural hair back into vogue with their afros, bushy twists, and pigtails it seems, and I'm glad to see it. A few of the new TV shows are employing a few young Black women sporting sexy, kinky hair. But I hope it's not just a temporary fad that will disappear with the show. Our natural hair is not a passing fad. It continually grows from our scalp whether relaxers are "in" or not; whether weaves are "in" or not, or whether pink, green or blue spikes are "in" or not. So, I want you to really begin to explore your hair, and perceive it differently. Think of it as normal hair, even if society doesn't. Go on and say it, "Yes, I have natural kinky hair, and I love it". As my sister friend from Detroit says, "Girl, let the kinks fly!".

Turn Kink Phobia into Kink Glory.

REGIONAL KINK PHOBIA

Some regions in this country tend to be less kink phobic than others, for instance, Black urban cities like New York, Chicago, or Detroit. Although you still have black or white mindsets that are inherently kink phobic, a city like New York is so crowded with mixtures, cultures, and styles from everywhere and all walks of life all milling together that people are somewhat sophisticated, tolerant, informed and cultivated about our natural hairstyles, more or less. Detroit is really a Chocolate City - enough said. I do find a lot of kink phobia in Los Angeles though, not necessarily in "the Hood", but Hollywood itself promotes kink phobia because of its nature. Hairdressers in L.A. know many incredible and highly skilled hair secrets for you to have the most expensive and gloriously straight hair there is, because that's what is in demand. Kinky hair is not generally promoted in L.A., except among "grass roots".

There's a lot of generational kink phobia also. And that's in any city. The youth are free-spirited, until they have to fit into the work world of older generations and parochial minded conservatives. Eventually, the youth turns to straight hair (to conform), and begin to experience all the problems therein of maintaining straight hair. It always looks nice at first. But eventually they succumb to the temptations for "short cuts" to straight hair, and all the problems inherent to maintaining that process.

CHAPTER 2

MAKING THE COMMITMENT TO GO NATURAL

"We teach you to love the hair God gave you."

Malcolm X

1925-1965

MAKING THE COMMITMENT TO GO NATURAL

Making the commitment to go natural or to cut out a relaxer is a difficult one for most Black women. Even making the decision to be *seen* without pressed or straightened hair is difficult. We literally have to overcome the fear of seeing our own hair first. Then we have to overcome the anxiety of the thought of styling our own "virgin" hair.

First of all, just overcoming the fear of seeing it is a big step. I had no idea exactly what three or four inches of my natural hair growth looked like.

Secondly, I had to overcome the fear and anxiety of attempting to style my natural hair. I had been so used to the hot irons and combs, I had no practice at styling my own natural hair since the days of the big Afro. I felt overwhelmed at the thought of dealing with my own hair.

I had to learn not to deal with my natural hair as if it was supposed to be straight. That's tough if you haven't been practicing with it for years. Occasionally, I would wear my relaxed hair blow dried without hot curling it. That's the roughest I would go and be seen, and even that is sporting a type of straight "processed" hair. Whenever the natural kinks and fuzz showed up, I would "touch-up" immediately with a mild relaxer.

DISASTERS TO REMEMBER

One day I decided to straighten it real silky. I bought SUPER. I assure you kink phobia had just taken my mind away from here. Do I need to describe what happened? PANIC! DISASTER!! I don't know what possessed me to put SUPER on top of my mild relaxer and my fine hair, except deep kink phobia. The only crazy answer I can begin to come up with is that I thought SUPER meant straighter.

Almost as soon as the SUPER relaxer cream went on top of my head, long thick tresses of my hair from the top of my head (where I was dumb enough to apply it) very easily slid off of my scalp into my hand.

"Oh No! Not again!"

Lucky for me I had some "stuff" handy that stopped breakage right away. I slopped it on. The hair immediately stopped breaking, and I somehow still had enough to hide the damage. Another beautiful head of hair gone because I wanted it straight, straight, straight. That was a horrible experience.

I remember once as a little girl, I decided to copy my Momma doing our hair and attempted to press my bangs, without permission. I was a kid fooling around in the kitchen where our hair got pressed. I decided my bangs would be straight forever if I just got the hotcomb red hot enough. Well, I did. The hair sizzled and melted off as soon as the burning red hot hotcomb touched my hair. Goodbye bangs.

I tried to comb more hair over the singed and burned out battleground hoping to camouflage the area so my mother would not notice it next time she combed my hair. Of course she noticed it right away.

"What did you do to your bangs?!" implored my mother.

"I tried to straighten my hair like you do".

After a proper scolding for touching a hot stove without permission, my mother comforted me, and told me she only used a *warm* comb, not a red hot burning one on my hair. Of course that would burn anyone's hair out, no matter how kinky or fuzzy their hair was. She was always assuring me that I had pretty hair. That's important to a young girl of color who's natural image is not necessarily revered in the movies at the Saturday afternoon cinema show.

Another time, many years later, trying to save money and avoid the hair salon now that I was living in a new city on my own, I went to a woman who did my hair privately. I really didn't know what she was doing, and she didn't know what she was doing. My hair looked beautiful for two days, then all of a sudden, when I dry combed it, I found lots of hair to be snapping off in the comb. I decided to wash it (as if that would help), and I experienced large handfuls of hair coming out wet in my hand. Girl. Now you know I was hysterical. I was crying so hard, my roommate at the time, gave me her hard earned $50 cash (which was a lot of money in the early 80's), and gave me the number of a "miracle worker beautician". Her girlfriend had very pretty hair and she swore by him.

I called him. It was late. I was in tears. "My hair...(sob, sob) ...it's coming out...(sob, sob) ...it's all wet...I can't stop it... I don't know what to do! (sob, sob, hysterical sob)..".

He told me his shop had been closed for hours, but he would meet me there ASAP and open it up for me.

"Thank you, (sob, sob). Thank you, I'll leave right now", I blubbered.

When I got there, he took one look, "Lord, what my Black women be doing to their hair", he sighed, as he started his magic.

I was sure I would have to sport a close cropped, shaved look. I was not really ready for that. I was traumatized.

That man was incredible. He saved my hair. He cut it to camouflage the damage (and it still bounced and flowed!), and he treated it once to twice per week for several weeks with an expensive repair solution. I worked my "temp" office job overtime to pay for it. Of course I stayed away from swimming pools. But when I left from that man's shop, I felt beautiful again.

Needless to say, he became my only beautician for the years I was around in town. He became my friend. Many years later, after

I had moved away and returned, he became my hairdresser on the TV show *"Roc"*. I was able to request him in my second season. Jerry Coke is the man for hair. My hair was "laying" on that show because of him and only him. He took care of my hair for many years until he became the most sought after and requested man in the business. He became so busy, he wasn't always available anymore after the show was canceled. I was happy for him though. I tried to bring him onto the film set of *"Set It Off"*, but there were schedule problems. And I experienced hair problems for the first time in many years because I didn't have someone whom I felt knew my hair. Although they were definitely competent and skilled professionals, I wanted Mr. Coke. One day I tried pressing my hair before I arrived at the set because I was always paranoid about new people handling my hair. I figured I would make it easy for them. I burned out a big chunk. Burned it right out. I tried to wear it "natural", but I was "directed" to wear it straight.

Then one day I was seduced by Rio. The so-called "no harsh chemical" relaxer which was being presented to us Black women through TV infomercials laced with lies (and lye). They even had someone appear to eat the stuff to prove there were no dangerous chemicals. What a crock of crap.

There were all kinds of class action lawsuits against Rio, but so what. They ripped us off and disappeared leaving Black women with broken hair and broken hearts.

This stuff was so insidious that it kept killing your hair for weeks - months. Once again, I was fortunate to have enough hair left to camouflage, but the damage was far reaching.

That was when I said "No more!". No more chemicals in my hair. Whether I applied it or a skilled professional applied it, I no longer wanted to *feel* dependent upon chemicals to feel good about my hair. I'd had it with promises of straight hair and empty "lyes". God grew beautiful hair out of my head (just like my Momma was always telling me). No, it's not straight, but in His wisdom He wanted it kinky, bushy, and thick. That was what I was going back to. ("Going back" - do you remember that term for pressed hair that reverts? - "it goes back". "Girl, I can't go swimming, my hair will go back"). And we know where it goes back to. Back to its natural African kinky state. So after one more hair disaster too many, I decided I'd rather have thick bushy hair rather than thin straight relaxed hair. And that's exactly what I was going to end up with if I kept after permanently straight hair.

Now, I realize us sisters all have different grades of hair. Some sisters have never had to see or feel a pressing comb because of a certain grade of hair. Some grades are kinkier and tighter than others, but still woolly. It is to the sister who knows the really woolly kink, and its effect on our society, that I hope to share this book with. This book is for you. For anyone else, maybe just a better understanding of an experience they are not necessarily subjected to.

I would love to see long braided or locked styles in conservative professions such as TV anchor women, Judges, or even First Class airline jobs, being able to be woolly-at-the-root if they choose, without being hassled, questioned, or fired. I would appreciate society not forcing us Black women to be afraid or repelled by our own hair. I wish long luscious kinks, locks, and braids to be just another hair style with no political or social judgment. A lot more Black women would wear them if it weren't for that job discriminating, anti-braids, anti-nap attitude. My Grandmother *finally* wanted braids one day, and sported them proudly around a few of her white senior citizen peers and heard "I don't like that". She was looking good too. But old neurotic hair attitudes accompanied with unsolicited rude remarks can be maddening.

But it also serves to consider that this "hair thing", not only with Black folks, but white folks as well, can be a very deep neurosis. I have often found myself wondering about the forefathers of this country and their wigged hairstyles, which I find mildly amusing.

What if society as we know it were reversed completely, and "our" nappy kinky woolly hair was considered normal, and white women spent their every grooming moment trying to keep straightness *out* of their hair, spending hours of curling it tighter and tighter and tighter. Hair that's meant to be straight or silky having to somehow alter its texture to be presentable to society on their jobs. Hair always being forced to do something it naturally does not want to do, scared it might revert to straightness. Then one day a woman says, "Enough, I'm wearing my hair straight", and she gets fired because that natural hair of hers offends society. The word "normal" would have an entirely different meaning for them.

Well, maybe that's a bit extreme but it's something close to what I have had to experience growing up in America. As a result of my experiences, I have had to reintroduce and reeducate myself to the real texture of my hair. I've had to learn it all over again. Changing the color of one's hair is not as difficult as maintaining another texture. In our society, straight silky hair is the "normal" desired hair texture to present, and it has caused me to lose more full heads of hair than I would have chosen in this life.

I have discovered to my pleasant surprise that I really find my natural hair texture to be very interesting and lovely. I wish I had given it a real chance decades ago. The many hair disasters, big and small, may have been non-existent. The myriad burns from curling irons, the tint/relaxer problems of dry breakage, the burning scalp tenderness after relaxer application, the attempts to "do" my hair myself, the short-short haircuts that I really didn't want at the time - all because I wanted and needed to have straight hair, for whatever reason, may not have been experienced.

Have you ever pressed your hair straight, danced at a party, and your hair puffs and swells looking nothing like it did when you left the house? Of course you have Sister. Or perhaps just go about your errands in humid weather, after you left your expensive hair salon, only to endure puff city? The hairstyle no longer looks attractive because it was styled to lay perfectly straight. The more you comb, the more it swells. And just forget the gym.

Humidity is no longer my sworn enemy. I can dance to a hot sweat, work out to a sweaty mess, and still walk away looking kinda cute. And of course with braids, there's not even a concern. You can walk in the rain or go swimming, and still look lovely and feel lovely. As long as our hair is clean, conditioned, and well-groomed, there is no reason for kink phobia.

HAIR TRANSITIONS

Weaves

I like weaves. They are incredibly skilled works of art, especially nowadays. They are extremely camouflaging and can provide the hair with a much needed rest because it's braided underneath and out of sight. If the hair that is used is the "fluff and go" type, it's real easy, making weaves a good choice for some ladies. Personally, I can only tolerate them temporarily like for a movie perhaps, but not as a regular style. I don't like the loss of control of my own hair. I don't like feeling dependent upon the professional to keep it looking tight. When they begin to grow out they must be dealt with right away, especially if it doesn't match your virgin hair texture (and it doesn't).

But if they work for you, be sure to get a good competent professional who will be available to the grow-out needs of your hair.

Oh, and did I mention, they are expensive. And if I'm going to wear a full head weave, I'm wearing the best hair money can buy.

Bonding

Personally, I trust nothing being glued to my hair. Eventual destruction is inevitable.

Braids

As I mentioned earlier, braids are my personal favorite grow-out aide. They are not necessarily the right choice for everyone, but for those that like them, I've dedicated an entire chapter on this style. (See Chapter on I LOVE BRAIDS).

One point of clarity I will mention here though is quality of hair. Although I recommend getting the expensive human hair for a weave, it's not always necessary for a hair transition using braids. The human hair is beautiful with relaxed hair, but you will still have the same grow-out problems of two different hair textures (especially if it gets wet). That is why under the Chapter on BRAIDS, I recommend the much less expensive synthetic for kinky hair. As more of your own fuzzy virgin hair reveals itself, the more those fuzzy braids will match your fuzzy hair, making it look all as one texture. This way it's easier to wear your own hair out with the braids unraveled on the ends. If your hair is naturally straight without much kink, human hair should be chosen for braids.

Locks

I recently saw a beautiful sister (a singer) who sported a head which was among the most beautiful locks I'd ever seen. They framed her lovely dark face with highlights of copper and auburn sprinkled with little brass beads. Being caught up in this hair book thing, I couldn't help but tell her how lovely her locked mane was. She thanked me and shared with me secretly that they were extensions. They were truly the first glorious locks I'd ever seen so perfectly *extended*. You know how closely us sisters can study that hair to see if it's real or not. The kinky hair absolutely matched her hair growing from her scalp in color and texture. It wasn't silky, curly or synthetic, but human kinky hair. She was so lovely. They were graceful and alive looking. She shared with me that it cost her $1,000.00, and that there was only one man in New York who does it. It's his technique alone. She flew there to have it done.

I shared with her my book writings. Of course we immediately bonded when I told her my title. She loved it. She shared with me the emotional hair problems that we sisters-of-the-nap seem to experience at some point and how greatly relieved she is now that her hair is no longer a problem of constant and anxious concern. She was allowing her own hair to lock underneath. I swear you could not tell where her hair ended and the locked extensions began. It looked as if it was all growing from her scalp. She told me that as she allows it to grow, she can eventually cut them off or just leave them in, never having to go to a short hairstyle. She preferred her face framed with hairlocks. She was a thing of alluring loveliness.

I think locks are beautiful if groomed and adorned. The politics that go along with locked hair is unfortunate for sisters because I'm sure more of us would sport them.

I'm not going to go into styling for locks here, of which there are many, but I will recommend reading books on hair locking like Nekhena Evans' book, if you are seriously considering that particular artform.

Haircut

Haircuts are the quickest way to eliminate a perm. I've had many haircuts. Some as a result of hair disasters, and some were my own trendy choice. But short haircuts are not necessarily desirable when your hair has been destroyed. You can either grow a relaxer out, or cut it all off. I prefer a gradual grow-out with braids, and snipping off the ends in between braid visits.

And let's face it. Short bald haircuts are not attractive on everyone. The bottom line is that if you want long, thick healthy hair, you have to work at it. It's worth it.

Hair transition decisions are difficult in the beginning after a disaster. One's self-esteem is injured. Panic has struck. The decision to go natural is usually after one disaster too many. And it's always met with the fear of, "What will I do with my hair?" That's the fear of the unknown: your own virgin hair.

Don't be affected by the comments made as you try different hairstyles involving a decision to deal with the kinks. We live in an anti-kink society. People will attack your nappiness whenever they can. Whites and Blacks. That's usually more of their own problem than it should be yours.

"Hey, your new hairstyle is lovely", never occurs to rude anti-braid and anti-kink people. They are too busy trying to impugn your dignity. Their choice of words will always be tinged with insult. From Whites it's usually laced with affirmations that it's not your *real* hair. But since they have discovered the existence of our extensions, a more enlightened white person will use that word, as they demand to know if it's yours. And by the way, your hair really does look good when they just have to ask. From some Blacks, believe it or not, it gets worse. You have to cringe at all the weave jokes the Black male comedians seem to revel in. The word "nappy" or "kinky" is always associated with some derogatory remark. Then, there are those women who just get jealous if you look too good. They're really going to find a remark to put your braids down. Stand up to it, and consider the source. You are going to get the silent treatment when your beautiful thick natural hair is revealed.

Don't take my word for it, do your own hair psyche experiments. If you are going through a hair transition, it can be really amusing and interesting. Sport a weave with straight hair and bouncy loose straight curls, and see for yourself how men respond. Then wear something short, tight, and kinky and see if you get a response. Wear red hair, blonde hair, short hair, or long hair. Test the attitudes of America for yourself. Straight hair vs. Kinky hair. It's a deep experience.

Good luck in making the decision to go natural. It's not just a hair change, it's a hair challenge.

CHAPTER 3

MAINTAINING NATURAL HAIR

"God made us his perfect creation. He made no mistake when he made us Black with kinky hair."

Marcus Garvey

1887-1940

MAINTAINING NATURAL HAIR

Okay, now you've got three years of new hair growth, and you are finally ready to stop braiding it. What to do now? Go back into a perm? Maintaining natural "virgin" hair is not as difficult as we are programmed to believe. As I have tried to emphasize, it's only difficult when we insist on dealing with it as if it is supposed to lay straight. Ideas of daily constant combing must change, if you are to cultivate your own natural hair. The "comb" as we know it, was not designed with natural Black hair in mind. We hopefully have established that.

You will have to invest in big wide tooth Afro piks for shampoo day (which I keep in the shower). But for daily grooming and maintenance, say goodbye to "the comb".

Daily grooming is done with your hands and fingers similar to the method described in Chapter 1 on "HAND GROOMING". Talk about going back to your primitive roots! I love styling my hair with my hands and a little conditioner, and zip - I'm gone. No more worry. No more comb-carrying, especially on those after-five evenings when you are all dressed up with that itty bitty little sparkly bag that won't fit a comb, a key, or anything else of importance.

It's takes a while to automatically stop grabbing that comb (out of habit), but I have found that I absolutely love experimenting and styling my hair this way. I like discovering which conditioners and groom-aides are now my favorite. The heavy emollient creams and oils that I wouldn't dare use on relaxed hair because they would weigh it down, are now perfect for my new naturally thick hair. I think you may be as pleasantly surprised as I was to find out how truly soft and pleasing to the touch your natural hair really is. But you have to give it a chance to grow out a few inches before you throw in the towel and go back to relax.

SHAMPOO

I always use a shampoo/detangler. The secret to not being overwhelmed by your thick head of bushy hair is keeping it untangled. By sectioning it off into large sections, and dealing with smaller amounts of hair at a time, the hair stays manageable and controllable. If you attempt to wash a head full of long thick bushy natural hair without softening it first, and sectioning it off into four or six large sections, you will be overwhelmed with kinkiness. "Oh, I have to relax this stuff", is all you will think. You will give up, saying it's too much work, it's too much time and energy. Who needs long hair anyway.

I always *pre*-shampoo my hair by conditioning it first. No, I don't just jump into the shower anymore. I would if it was straight or short but, we don't deal with our hair like it's straight anymore right?). So, I pre-shampoo (or soften) my hair with a thick conditioner like raw African Shea Nut butter, or a good detangling cholesterol creme (like Lustrasilk). Apply it to dry hair, because the point is to soften and detangle it first with your fingers so you can gently comb it out with a wide tooth comb or afro pik, and section it off into big fat braids (or use hair clips). This puts it into an easy untangled and manageable state before you shampoo.

Actually shampoo each section separately, and fat-braid it back up out of the way of the other sections. With your wide-tooth afro pik, comb the hair through while washing it, keeping it untangled. That's the key to keeping the tangledness to a minimum, actually combing it out loosely while shampooing it in sections.

CONDITIONER

I condition in the exact same pattern as I shampoo, in sections, combing through and "fat-braiding" the hair back up as I go, using intense creme and oil conditioners.

Hot oil treatments are great whenever you want to spend the extra time pampering your ever growing thick new hair. Olive oil, jojoba oil, even plain vegetable oil are good ingredients to use. You can either sit in the hot California sun, or under a hair dryer for about ten to 15 minutes, then rinse.

Don't ever be afraid to condition and rinse twice (especially if you have the time). It only makes natural hair more manageable, soft, and ultimately luxurious.

I *always* use a leave-in conditioner when I am through with the rinse-out conditioners.

One good advantage to going natural is the elimination for the need to buy the super expensive specialized conditioner products to meet the specific needs of relaxed hair. Have you ever noticed all of the products for relaxed hair care that have emergency and corrective-to-damage type names? That's because eventually your relaxer is going to be in trouble. They count on that.

For natural virgin hair, any basic good creme conditioner of your choice will do. They generally don't cost as much as the specialized conditioners for processed hair.

Another advantage is that when you travel you don't have to look for that one section in the back of the store on the bottom shelf for Black Hair Care, as if we just are not part of mainstream America. Black hair care stores are great, but it's a mighty big world out there, and if you travel around the world or just to a lot of cities in this country alone, you may not always have the convenience of finding that specialized hair product. With natural virgin hair, any emollient super-detangling cream will do. Just remember the thick rich creams are preferred to handle thick kinky hair. The light watery lotions for relaxed hair are no longer as effective for natural hair (except the "leave-in" conditioners). There are always plenty of spray detanglers on the shelf. If I'm out-of-town and I find myself buying a non-generic type detangler, I purchase a little moisturizing hair oil and add a capful or two to the solution. That's if my regular products are not available.

COMB-OUT

This is usually where the faint of heart will make excuses for wearing very short cropped hair, or just the heck with it and get a perm. But it doesn't have to be that way. Comb-out should not be difficult if you have followed the pre-shampoo, wash, and condition steps I've described.

After I put my leave-in conditioner into my hair, I "fat-braid" it back up into large sections. Depending on the style I want, I either begin to twist it at this point while very wet, or, I comb out each section with a spray detangler, fat-braid it back up, and let it dry a little under a dryer, but not bone dry. It will still be pliable and supple if it stays a little damp. Then you are ready for styling by setting it with twists, or you can blow-dry it out if you must. Frizz Ease makes an excellent Corrective Styling Gel perfect for applying to wet, damp, or dry twists.

If you still have relaxer on the ends, they will be extremely tangly with both textures of hair to deal with, so take extra care to remove the tangles *with your fingers.*

Surprisingly, this entire shampoo, condition, and comb-out process becomes easier. The longer the hair gets, the fewer "fat-braid" sections are needed, and the easier it is to detangle with a wide-tooth comb, always starting at the ends of the hair first, working your way up to the scalp.

This is basically the only day you will concern yourself with actually combing the hair. You no longer comb for daily style. You comb to gently detangle the hair while it's soft, supple, and freshly conditioned on shampoo day.

DRYING YOUR NATURAL HAIR

Dry naturally whenever possible. Hot arid California weather is great for drying virgin hair naturally. But for those "back east" in heavy winters and moist, cold weather, of course, you must speed the drying process up artificially.

Blow-drying natural hair can be done, and is a convenient option. We are not going for straight hair, just *stretched* hair. (We used to call it "afro blow-out"). At this point, you can rub a good heat protector product, or just a little oil throughout the hair before blow-drying. Dry one, small, easy section at a time. Gently stretch the hair out with a wide tooth attachment, and then "big-braid" or "fat-braid" that section out of the way. Of course, the big braid will be longer after it's stretched.

The other option is to sit your entire head under a hood-type dryer after the hair is braided up into fat sections, then proceed to twist. This way a lot of the heavy, excess water will begin to dry at the scalp area. Hood dryers are a good investment, because they gently dry the hair evenly, eliminating the risk of heat damage, that may happen with a blow dryer.

STYLING YOUR NATURAL HAIR

Twists

I'm still amazed discovering the myriad styles I can get with twists. I find that the same time it takes to blow-dry, press, and hot curl, I've twisted my hair and allowed it to dry.

Twists are simply done with a thick, alcohol-free gel. The thing that is really important to remember with this style is that the thicker and kinkier the hair, the more you must be sure to completely coat the hair with the gel. Coat each lock of hair as you twist. The hair must be completely dry before releasing them otherwise they will not set properly. As you twist the gel-coated hair, actually pull and stretch the hair as you twist. You must apply a generous amount. Don't skimp. Don't be afraid to really coat the hair as long as the gel is alcohol-free. It will only damage your hair if you attempt to *comb* it afterward.

I either let the twists hang, or, I ponytail them back with a scrunchy band, and dry it that way for a relaxed twist look. Sometimes I put on a nylon stocking cap and dry it that way for a flatter look. I can elect to leave the twists in for one look, or unfurl them for another look. The important thing to remember for this style is that the hair must be completely dry before untwisting it in order for the curls and waves to set.

Once it's set, you don't use a comb again to maintain the style. As a matter of fact, you don't use a comb again until shampoo time. You can "re-set" a twist with a quick-set gel at any time before shampoo day.

Once I've worn the unraveled twists for a few days, I constantly add a conditioner to the curly ends, either a gel, cream, or pomade. I find that the African kinky hair-ends love this constant moisture replenishment. My hair is thicker and longer than I could ever get it to grow in a traditional afro where the ends were always naturally dry because the hair was being combed or "picked" away from the scalp.

Another style to try is blow-drying and stretching it out first, then twist, and dry again. You get a glistening rich texture to your natural hair. But if you twist after blow-drying, make sure you lay the gel on extra thick, making sure your hair really is bone dry when you untwist them, otherwise the waves will "crawl" back up not setting properly. The released twists have actually "wet-set" your hair texture into crisp little waves. You can let them hang, or upsweep and pin the hair into many attractive styles until the next shampoo. As long as you *don't comb them out,* those beautiful natural springy waves are set and easy to maintain even in humidity.

There's no discernible texture change in the hair even if it does puff up. It actually looks full and lovelier when it puffs up.

Something else very important that I discovered one day while removing the twists was that I shouldn't start from the bottom up to remove them. It takes a lot of time and actually destroys the style. I could untwist faster and easier by rubbing the dry twist first with a little hairdressing, and untwist from top to bottom in one easy pull motion. If it tangles on the way down, stop, rub a little extra oil, and continue. It will slide apart with wave-curl intact. If you wish the curls to hang a little looser, make sure to use a non-water base hair-dressing, otherwise the hair will draw back up. But even that's okay, because with this style water is not the enemy. Raw shea butter is perfect, or just plain hair grease. It actually stretches the hair out.

The very short twists on me were not my preference, so I waited until my natural hair had grown about four inches in length before I started sporting the twists. It was at that length that I had to figure out something to do with my hair.

You can easily wear the twists under hats and scarves which also help the twists to lay flat and loose. At night, I tie it all back with several scrunchies. I like sleeping that way. (Remember the days of sleeping with rollers in your hair? Hard rollers? The things we do.) Just remember you are styling and grooming with your hands each day, not a comb.

I wish I had discovered this easy way to deal with my hair many years ago, instead of feeling my feminine beauty was dependent upon chemical relaxers and pressing combs. Now, I only press my hair with a warm electric comb for a once-in-a-while temporary change to stretch the hair out (not bone strait press it), and never on a rainy day. When relaxed or pressed hair bushes up in wet weather, it looks as if you've lost the hairstyle to bad weather. With rain, relaxed curls look flat, limp, and frizzy; straightened "virgin" hair looks completely "gone-back"; and a twisted natural style just becomes fuller, curlier, and lovelier. It doesn't look so obvious like

I lost my hair-do. If I lived in Seattle (where it rains all the time it seems), I would literally donate all of my pressing combs and hot curling tools to the African American Hair History Museum, my point being that I would never attempt to press and curl in rainy or humid weather if it were not absolutely necessary. I would just enjoy wearing my own natural hair.

Although "afros" are making a lovely come-back, there are other styles that African hair can be worn in which actually help and allow the American-African hair to grow longer. Yes, I said American first. Our American kink has been mixed with many, many hair types in this country of ours. Our kink has many different and varying degrees of tightness and curl. The haircare I share with you here is especially for that mixture of hair. We have African kink at the roots, but we are not African citizens, no matter how kinky ones' hair may, or may not be. We are Americans with varying degrees of kinky African hair. Back in the original day of the "afro", we as Black people were just beginning to even reveal our natural hair texture. An "afro" or "natural" was the only style we really knew to do with that natural hair.

My sister has that crawly "good-stuff" which never really needed a pressing comb. Amazingly, I got the "Twists" idea from her. She took the time to twist her beautiful crawly hair one day before our Thanksgiving Dinner, and in no time really, she had lovely twist-locks. I tried it a little at a time as I removed a few braids (in the bangs section only), and experimented with small amounts of hair at a time. I discovered that my kinky stuff did the same thing her crawly stuff did. After all, she's of African ancestry too.

Nowadays, there are many great styling aide products that address the needs of our natural hair. Products labeled for twists, locks, braids, and even "kinky" hair; even products that specialize in removing locks and knots.

Braids and natural hair make our life easy, but Kink Phobia won't give us a rest. Kink Phobia won't allow us the dignity of being ourselves. That is why a lot of us have no current experience in styling our natural hair. It's always approached from a negative perspective, as if something is wrong or unfinished because the hair is in that kinky state, but given half of an aesthetic chance, long, twisted, kinky hair is soft, beautiful, and an attractive crowning glory on the sister sporting it.

NO COMB

By deciding to wear your hair in it's most natural form, our entire relationship with "the comb" has to change.

Have you ever wondered why people with locks can grow their hair so very long? No matter how tight the kink? It's because they are no longer *combing* the hair. Our hair is meant to be styled and cared for with our hands.

Extra-wide tooth combs, good quality afro piks, and "lifters", are necessary to invest in, but the idea of daily combing is no longer necessary for styling. For the **"no comb look",** you simply style with conditioner or hairdressing on the hands, and pull, massage, and sculpt the hair until it falls attractively around your crown, grabbing large sections, gently stretching it out more and more, making it full, kinky curly, and lovely, allowing it to go or fall wherever it pleases. Specifically, you are not running your fingers through the hair (as if it were silky straight), but rather on the hair. This way the kinky waves and curls stay set. If you comb, you comb them out to frizz, and you tear your hair out. That is why you use your hands. By styling your hair this way during the week before you shampoo again, the hair rests, thickens, and grows as if it was up in braids. And let me tell you, it gets real liberating not always having to carry a comb.

Sometimes, for a change, I wear it stretched out with the blow-dryer after shampoo, and perhaps an electric comb pressed through the finished style. I might twist it up a day or so later, (see photos). For that style, it's necessary to carry an afro pik or wide tooth comb, and give it a little combing care whenever you feel the need, always combing the ends out first. If you rub the hair-ends between your fingers, it will loosen any curly tangles for the pik to comb through, not snatch out. Be firm but gentle when combing your hair always. Don't let impatience cause you to carelessly rake a pik through your scalp. If you want luscious thick hair you must begin to treat it with patience and care.

With virgin hair, the electric pressing comb is not going to get hot enough to damage the hair or even <u>straighten</u> the hair, it will only stretch it out giving it length. Always press with a good hairdressing. I always apply a good light hair oil and a thermal protector. It keeps the hair well conditioned.

To maintain the style each day, I just tie the hair back in a ponytail scrunchy at night, or now that my hair is really long, I line several scrunchies up in one long kinky ponytail overnight. The next day I just pull it out with my hands and I'm good to go. No comb.

TEXTURIZERS/RELAXERS/CURLY PERMS

New relaxers are on the market these days. It seems they will never go completely out of style or away from our dependence on them.

Some relaxers have lye base, some are no-lye. They all still have a chemical of some sort to permanently alter the hair texture. You are still dependent upon expensive specialized conditioners, and professional hair salon visits to apply and maintain it.

Texturizing is really a very mild relaxer applied once in a while to <u>loosen</u> the tight kinky curl only, not severely straighten it. This is not so damaging because you're not striving to keep it straight by re-applying it every month with "touch-ups". I know a few sisters who are sporting texturized hair, and have better hair for it. Some don't. One sister, I know, said she wished she had stayed chemical-free and not put it in her natural hair at all. By the way, my mother is a licensed cosmetologist. She too has always had hair that grew fast as weeds. She always took excellent, outstanding care of my hair when I was a child, as well as her own. I didn't start having hair problems until I moved away and began experimenting as an adult with different promises and products without consulting her. Even with a texturizer, my hair was regularly maintained by a professional - my mother.

Curly perms or jheri "scary" curls are really passe. We all remember the hilarious scene in the movie where the guy begged for his curl activator on his knees. Did we really go through that stage? We wanted loose-looking straight curls so bad we suffered through the Jheri curl, with grease dripping in droplets everywhere. Natural hair absorbs nutrient oils; processed hair does not. It sits on top of the hair scaring anyone who comes near it. When it gets old, the frizzy, brittle, unmanageable hair is awful, and you regret putting that stuff in your hair. To remove it, you must cut. You cannot put any other chemical process on top of it without losing it altogether. The wet curl, the dry curl - it was all bad. I watched my fellow sisters suffer with that perm and I was glad I hadn't succumbed to that temptation.

TINTS/DYES/HIGHLIGHTS

Tints, dyes, and highlights are potentially disastrous with perms. At first, done professionally, they look gorgeous. But haven't you ever wondered where that hair slowly disappears to? Without vigilant professional care and condition, it will break, and slowly disappear, or become hopelessly dull, dry, and unmanageable. Even with the deep conditioning treatments, you will constantly be told to "clip those fried ends" til you clip it away. It probably won't grow faster than the every 2-3 weeks of end-clipping, so it appears your hair is not really growing past a certain length. Well, you're probably clipping away a good inch every time you re-color which is probably often, so a colored shorter style is what you are reckoned with.

I actually use lemon juice to highlight my hair. I've used instant type highlighteners with the sun on the natural highlights in my own hair, on selected strands, but be careful. You don't want to spray all over. It can have an adverse effect even on strong natural hair if you spray too much too often without intense conditioners. Spray it on relaxed hair, and you can say goodbye to those strands after a few shampoos.

Hennas are natural extracts. They are not damaging to the hair but they are not as dramatic in change or permanency either. You can't really get blonde highlights if desired either. You get more red.

And of course no one can blame you for rinsing out the gray. As a matter of fact, blonde highlights tend to cover gray hair just fine. It doesn't stand out as much when it grows back, and a lot of sisters of different complexions are playing around with the honey blonde shades freely, and quite sucessfully, nowadays. But I must admit, I've seen some sisters who maintain gray or white-silver hair and it looks beautiful on those gray foxes. I've even seen gray braids and extensions that I thought were absolutely lovely, and completely undetectable.

So, let's recap this section for clarity of hair handling:

- *pre*-shampoo (condition dry hair), rinse
- shampoo, condition again, rinse
- fat-braid and comb-out, in sections
- twist
- dry
- (option: unfurl dried twists)

-or-

- *pre*-shampoo (condition dry hair), rinse
- shampoo, condition again, rinse
- fat-braid in sections
- blow-dry (stretching hair)

- o twist (with gel)
- o dry again
- o unfurl dried twists for luscious style & shine

Just remember, caring for natural hair means conditioning it before you shampoo. Hot oil or cream conditioner should be applied to dry hair for super absorption and easy handling before you shampoo.

FALLING IN LOVE

Well, here we are. It's a new millennium and I feel as if I have just now discovered with appreciation the true nature of my hair, even though I lived through the "I'm Black and I'm Proud" era. And I really love it.

It's difficult not succumbing to the pressures to relax either from associates or advertising temptations. Everyone in America feels that straight hair is the "norm". Unfortunately, we Black people still subscribe to that archaic way of thinking too. But there are those who are enlightened, and happier for it.

I remember in the 70's when I first went "natural" and my sweet grandmother was upset that I "messed up" all my pretty hair that my mother slaved over to grow. All her friends were upset as well. I remember how unsure I was about unveiling my new hairdo, (the big "Afro"), to my father. How surprised and relieved I was when he told me he liked it. My enlightened father was part of that movement. I don't think I could have continued to sport my "fro" (as we called it) without his genuine approval. But this Black man loved my Black hair; it made all the difference in truly understanding what we as a people were experiencing. We were falling in love with ourselves, our hair, our nose, our "natural" selves.

The "fro" was a defining, yet somewhat confining style for some, and the 80's saw the return of the relaxer. I succumbed as well seeking convenience and versatility, but ironically, I have found that now, after rediscovering the true beauty of the kink.

Braids and kinks in this American society tend to be associated (consciously or unconsciously) with negativity. The music videos seem to be the only place left for true Black hair liberty. How ironic when it was not always that way. Just research the styles worn by black artists in the 40's, 50's, and early 60's. There was not a strand of nappy hair - anywhere. Not a kink if they could help it. Not even James Brown himself, until *"Say It Loud"*.

CHAPTER 4

TRIBUTE TO THE PIONEERS

"Who taught you to hate the texture of your hair?"

Malcolm X

1925-1965

TRIBUTE TO THE PIONEERS

(Angela Davis, Rosalind Cash, and Whoopi Goldberg)

I would be remiss if I didn't single out strong beautiful Black women who braved the early days of letting the kinks fly. These particular Black women influenced my own hair embracement of kink glory.

Angela Davis

Angela Davis was, for me, the first paradigm of kinky glory because of her beauty and media profile. The last photo I saw of her in a woman's magazine, she was sporting thick natural woolly waves and kinks. Still beautiful. I proudly wore my "Angela Davis 'fro'", when I took my high school graduation photo. Those of us who sported afros thought Angela Davis' hairstyle was the role model. During her troubles, she was actually able to move through society with her hair straightened, and remained unrecognized for a while because she was not wearing her famous "afro". At one time white folks seemed to only see us by our hair. The Afro was a symbol of sorts to label us. They never really understood what wearing our natural hair meant to us. They still don't really. Angela Davis never succumbed back to the pressures of society to relax. During the late 80's I saw a photo of her with glorious long locks in the beautiful picture book, *"I Dream A World"* by Brian Lanker.

Thank you Angela Davis for paving the way to Black hair enlightenment.

Rosalind Cash

This woman is extraordinarily special to me. I had the great privilege and experience of working with her and knowing her, however brief. She was cast to play my mother on *"Roc"* in all her hairlocked glory. This is another sister who never succumbed back to relaxers once she went natural.

And in the early 90's, you just did not see any Black women on television in long glorious locks.

After *"Roc"*, she got a contract on ABC's *"General Hospital"*. I called her. I was so excited and happy for her and the fabulous role she played on the show. She was teaching them to deal with her locks, and she wore them pinned up in beautiful sculptured styles. I often wished they would let her wear them down her back, but I think they were afraid of her looking too young when she was playing a woman much older.

Finally I got to see those gorgeous sandy brown and gray locks flow in *"Tales From The Hood"*, (one of my favorites). Her role was great, her hair glorious, her acting exquisite.

She told me once, "It takes a lot of courage to stop putting a comb in your hair. People don't like it".

Roz was beautiful and I miss her terribly, although her beautiful image, her gentle spirit, and courage is forever with me. Thank you Roz.

Whoopi Goldberg

It almost seems as if we've never seen Whoopi without locks.

I recall when she sort of braided herself into locks. There was an outpouring from Blacks (above all people) who didn't like it. I didn't even know the woman, but I was offended by the constant digs at her chosen hairstyle.

Well, thanks to Whoopi, there are a few more pretty sisters wearing locks on TV and film. Whoopi's glorious career has done a lot to help that. She is a world renown movie star, and her image has allowed other hairlocked beauties to at least have a slight chance in the film and TV industry.

Thank you Whoopi Goldberg.

Even though I know there are a lot more pioneers who braved the early struggles of wearing natural kinky hair, these are just three who greatly influenced my path. I know there are plenty of sisters that come to mind when you think about it.

There's the attractive Black teacher in high school who wore a "natural", and because she was so beautiful, intelligent, respected, and liked - no one dared to attempt to fire her.

There's my beautiful cousin who sported a "natural" into "locks" when the rest of us was still "tripping" on braids. She has luscious long thick hair that has grown for many years. I remember when her hair "wouldn't grow" because of relaxers and hot combs. Now, she doesn't even own a comb.

CLOSING THOUGHTS

Just think of how courageous a woman of color has to be just to exist in America in all her nappy glory.

Hair care, because of Black women is a multi-million dollar business. It needs us, to need it, to wear our hair straight, and to keep our hair straight. Those professionals that braid and lock are usually separate from those that relax and press. My hair is much thicker and healthier now than it ever was with chemicals and hot curls. So for the naysayers who say this is not true, the proof is my healthy, thick, soft natural hair.

Everything natural about us seems somehow problematic for America, and at one time was actually viewed as abhorrent.

Everything naturally African by nature in this country has been distorted, insulted, and made fun of (in American movies and cartoons), or it has been suppressed, or altered in some way to not reflect who we are, and we are very sensitive to it. Our hairstyles have been insulted, and even worse, forbidden. Even we, as blackfolks, have dread of our own hair, and our own nappy "kitchen". (Did you just toot a familiar hoot at that term?) For those readers who may be unfamiliar with that term, it refers to the curly little nap balls at the nape of the neck. When you start to sweat your pressed hair out in a hot heated kitchen, those cute kinky little fuzz balls let people in the South know just how much kink (or African) you had in your blood. Once again, our natural hair was a condition of shame lored over us to determine our "breeding", or bloodline status of some sort. Those that had no "kitchen", whose hair fell flat on their neck, were "better". Light or dark was also an issue, but could sometimes take a back seat to "good hair", when it came to desirability. If you were light with straight falling hair, (no "kitchen" on your neck), you could literally pass for white, or "exotic" something, anything, but colored.

Why write about this aspect of our hair trials? We must tell it to document and share our common understanding and experiences in American culture. No one can tell it, but us, as we know it to be. My passion for writing this book is to hopefully inspire and enrich the self-esteem of my fellow kinky haired comrades. The feeling that comes over you when you wear your natural hair, and *know* that you are beautiful and desirable, is close to an epiphany for us sisters.

The pressure and desire to conform to straight hairstyles is ever present, but even that is slowing making a turn. There is a bit more relaxation over naps than it used to be. I know I am happier with my natural hair. My husband is happier with my lush woolly hair. He's thinks it's sexy, and loves touching it. I prefer the bushy feel of my thick hair now, opposed to the thin feel of my relaxed hair. I even get a lot of compliments and admiring head turns, from blacks and whites. Some women just look on in envy, and some really want to know how to do that with their own hair, and how can I possibly live without a perm? Oh, and by the way, I've even discovered that I actually do have "hair that moves!", after all.

Now, I know a lot of sisters will think that I am lightskinned, so I must have a certain fair grade of hair. Absolutely not true. Kink is kink. I've broken a few combs myself. The basic properties of kink-and-curl are present no matter how tight your naps may be. I tried my hair method on a pretty ebony skinned sister, with the tightest kink. She insisted that this would not work for her hair, and that she absolutely *hated* her hair. (And I sympathized with her, because I used to *hate* my hair). She had a very thick amount of short hair which she wore in a tight, firm, bushy natural. She half-heartedly tried it, not sticking to the instructions I laid out for her. She ended up with frizz, because she took them out incorrectly. I personally twisted her hair myself, making sure it was absolutely dry, before removing the twists, *properly*. It did my heart so much good to see the unbridled joy on her face when she saw her tight African nap transformed into natural, beautiful twists and corkscrew curls.

"You mean I can do this to my entire head!?, she exclaimed.

"All you have to do is take the time", I grinned back at her, sharing the memory of the joy I felt when I first discovered the many intricate twists and twirls I could achieve in my hair without heat or chemicals. She was amazed at how long and soft her natural kinky tress really was. Another benefit is that this style actually softens the hair over time, allowing it to grow long and strong.

It's really not that our hair "won't grow", it's just what we do to it once it's there that makes it seem as if it does not grow for some sisters. If you shave your head bald, your hair will grow back, you cannot stop it. So, your hair grows. By not combing it all of the time to groom it, but yet addressing the needs of natural dryness in the kinky hair, it won't disappear. The one understanding I acquired after reading *"Good Hair"*, was to stop combing my hair, and wear it in styles which emphasize it's natural kink-and-curl qualities. I began to really experiment and discover easy ways of dealing with my hair that really are not difficult. As a matter of fact, I don't wish for straight silky hair anymore. I prefer my own. It may take a little more time on shampoo day, but while it's being attractively styled without the comb throughout the week, the hair is thickening and growing longer. It's not being pulled, snatched, or burned out everyday. The longer the kinky hair is allowed to naturally grow, the easier it is to handle, even on shampoo day.

Not all hair methods are right or comfortable for everyone. The idea of not using a comb for daily styling is unimaginable to some, *("No comb?! Girl, are you crazy?!"),* and may take some getting used to, but there are some of us who fall into the kink category, who have certain unique needs in natural hair care that isn't always available or even commercially-celebrated knowledge, if you choose not to wear it straight. A healthy head of strong virgin hair may not ever really want to see a curling iron again. If you choose to wear it chemically straight, always let a licensed professional apply it. Leave the TV infomercial ads alone! But, if you are ready for true hair independence, with control and variety of style over your own kinky hair, then give it a brave try. I hope you don't lose your job, or your patience, but give it a chance. You may never recoil from the word "kinky" or "nappy" to describe your beautiful hair again, but actually revel in it. Yes, your arm muscles will get worked dealing with your new thick virgin hair, and it may take a little more feminine time, but you just might discover, as I did, that your own natural, nappy, knotty, kinky, fuzzy, woolly hair is really very beautiful, and well worth it. By experimenting with it this way, you may even discover certain characteristics which are unique only to our kinky hair, that make you fall in love with it. That's what I discovered along my journey through this Black woman's hair.

"The more blackness a woman has, the more beautiful she is."

Alex Haley

1921 - 1992

BIBLIOGRAPHY

Brittenum-Bonner, Lonnice - *Good Hair: For Colored Girls Who've Considered Weaves When The Chemicals Became Too Ruff,* Crown Publishers 1992.

Evans, Nekhena - *Everything You Need To Know about Hairlocking,* second edition, New Being' Enterprises, A&B Books, 1994.

Lanker, Brian - *I Dream A World,* Stewart, Tabori & Chang, Inc. 1989.

Kathy Russell, Midge Wilson, Ronald Hall - *The Color Complex*, Doubleday Publishers 1992.

Griffin, John Howard - *Black Like Me*, New American Library, Penguin Putnam, Inc. 1962.

Haley, Alex -*The Autobiography of Malxolm X*, The Ballantine Publishing Group 1964.

Newman, Richard - *African American Quotations,* The Oryx Press, Checkmark Books 2000

PHOTOGRAPH CREDITS: Dan Martin, Alan Weissman, Martin, Mr. & Mrs. Hoye, and friends.

Front Cover Photo and Back Cover Photo: Dan Martin

PRODUCTS FOR VIRGIN HAIR

The following is a suggested list of products I have found especially beneficial and softening for virgin hair manageability. One of the great advantages to washing your hair in sections, is that you can use different products on different sections of the hair and feel for yourself which ones are especially beneficial for the needs of your own hair. Some actually soften, condition, and detangle the hair almost as soon as you apply it. Some work remarkably well with heating caps. You will discover products that meet the specific needs of your own hair once you start experimenting with natural hair. Just remember any product with water will soften and draw the hair back up; any product with oil base will soften and stretch the hair out.

Most of the products I have mentioned are very affordable at any hair supply store, and some can be found in regular drugstores. The ones that are especially expensive, I have made note of it. Remember sometime superior products may always cost a little more, but your hair is worth it, and the ability and freedom to style and maintain it yourself.

All products are not right for everyone's kinks, these are just a few I've had good results with, so have fun trying different ones until you find what's just right for your own tight curly tangles. Just remember, our natural hair has a different feel and different needs than our relaxed hair.

Pre-Shampoo Cream with Shea Butter (creme nourrissante au beurre de karite) J. F. Lazartigue (Paris)

Extremely expensive, and you may have to special order from a Beauty/Hair Supply store. Leaves hair amazingly soft before you shampoo. Sometimes, I leave on overnight under a conditioning cap, and shampoo in the morning for extra deep conditioning. Outstanding product.

Lustrasilk Cholesterol Creme Conditioner Super Detangling Formula

For me this is the absolutely *best priced* and highly *effective conditioner* for natural virgin hair on the market. I'm almost afraid to print it in fear they may realize what they have and raise their price. It's a superior detangling cream for removing braids, as well as maintaining virgin hair. The price is amazingly cheap compared to some expensive products I've used that are not as effective. I get even more superior results if I use a heating cap, although it's not necessary. Excellent stuff.

3-n-1 Plus Dark 'N Lovely Detangling Conditioning Shampoo

Although there are many combination shampoo/conditioners on the market, I find this one to be a consistently great shampoo for thick unruly hair. Keeping natural hair from getting overly tangled is the key. Modest price. Affordable.

Dark 'N Lovely Restore & Repair Reconstructive Hair Therapy Creme

It comes in a small jar, and is superior for maintaining natural hair. I experienced a little blow-dryer damage once and found this creme especially soothing for the abused hair. Watch that blow dryer! Modest price.

Dudley's Hair Rebuilder

This product was especially effective after my Rio damage. After several uses there was a real permanent improvement in the condition of my hair. A bit expensive, but worth it.

Frizz Ease Corrective Styling Gel

This product is absolutely essential for "California Twists". It softens, smoothes, and actually stretches and sets the hair without alcohol. It seems to improve the condition of the hair. Better yet, it comes in a most convenient slim stand-up pump, making it real easy to dispense while twisting the hair. It's usually in any drugstore or grocery market, and it is not terribly expensive. It's a superior gel. I lay it on very thick and, of course, never comb the hair after it's set with this gel. It sets crisp pretty little waves once you remove the twists.

Mink Oil Gel
by African Royale distributed by Bronner Bros. Atlanta

This gel is also superior for twists. As an added benefit it softens and conditions the hair leaving it amazingly soft to touch and pretty to look at. It takes a little longer to completely dry because of all of the emollients penetrating the hair, but it is worth it for the glistening healthy shine afterward. It is not terribly expensive either. Quite reasonable. I highly recommend this wonderful product for Ella's "California Twists". Lay it on thick.

Daily Doctor
by African Royale

An effective liquid leave-in conditioner which makes hair immediately manageable and soft. It helped with my blow-dryer damage, so that I didn't have to cut the abused hair off.

M.O.M. (Miracle Oil Moisturizer)
by African Royale

Exquisite oil moisturizer for natural hair that needs taming. Very rich and emollient; not too expensive.

Soft Sheen Breakthru Anti-Breakage Everyday Moisturizer; Shampoo; and Deep Intense Conditioner by Optimun Care

This is an amazing new trio on the market. It actually does what it advertises doing. It *stops* breakage. It actually checks those curly strands of hair that seem to keep coming out when you wash or handle the hair. Sometimes I mix the moisturizer with some of my other favorite products to make my own custom hairdress, or setting gel. I highly recommend all three of these products for natural hair maintenance. This line also makes a great heat protectant for blow-drying. I find the price varies depending on what neighborhood you are in when you purchase it, but generally affordable.

Nexxus Headress Leave-In Conditioner

I put this on wet or dry hair. Expensive, but excellent.

Nexxus Designing Butter High Fashion Texture Creme

Very emollient for natural hair. Very expensive.

Doo Gro Stimulating Growth Oil; Deep Down Intense Penetrating Conditioner; and Growth Repair Conditioner

This company seems to be making excellent products for natural hair. The Growth Repair Conditioner is very effective. The Stimulating Growth Oil is great for all around use including hot oil treatment, blow-dry, or a light press. It can also be added to a weak conditioner or shampoo for added benefits. The Intense Penetrating Conditioner is super softening. Excellent products, affordable price.

Paul Mitchell Super-Charged Conditioner Super Moisturizer

Sometimes I use this luxurious product as a last creme rinse on my natural hair. It's very expensive, but well worth it for the manageability and softness of your hair. One of my favorites. Easy to find, especially in general Beauty Hair Supply stores.

St. Ives Revitalizing Conditioner and St. Ives Hair Repair (Intensive Conditioning Treatment)

Although it says conditioner, I occasionally use it as a last rinse. Effective and inexpensive. Easy to find.

Parnevu Leave-In Creme Hairdress, and Leave-In Conditioner for Dry Hair

This product I found was especially helpful when I was coming out of my braids and making the attempt to begin to wear natural hair. Use sparingly. Price is moderate, and you have to find it at hair and beauty supply stores.

New Image - Damage Free - Thermal Active Conditioning Styler

Absolutely great product. Apply before blow-drying. Modest price.

Thermal Prep (Heat Protection, Level 3); and Thermal Finish (Thermal Curling Mist) by Kizure - Thermal Kontrol Options

For those times that I want to stretch the hair out with a blow dryer or electric comb, I found these products to work wonders in protecting the hair. Price is a little more than moderate, but worth it.

Sheenique Botanical Potion (Wearable Treatment) by Summit Laboratories, Inc.

I find this to be an absolutely superior product for wearing twists. Can be hard to find, but the price is right.

Kemi-Moyst L.I.C. (Leave In Conditioner)

Excellent product. Leaves braids especially smelling wonderful. Hard to find. Price is moderate.

Miss Cool 5 Minute Fast Set by Soft Sheen

Great for re-setting twists in between shampoos. Good price.

Shea Butter by ORGANIC Root Stimulator "Softening" Hair & Scalp Lotion

Great for twists, braids and kinks. Moderate price.

Allways Natural Indian Hemp Conditioning Hair Dress

Excellent no-water base pomade. Smells nice. Inexpensive.

Royal Crown Indian Sage

Gelatinous and rich no-water base pomade. Smells good. Inexpensive. (Been in Black households for years).

Raw African shea butter

This you must find in Black Beauty/Hair Care stores, or African markets and festivals. It is a hardened cream in its' raw form. You may add a few drops of your favorite essential oil to help soften the butter and add aroma. Clove, sandalwood, or vanilla are my favorite scents to add. You must smear it between your fingers before applying to your dry hair or twist. Just coat the hands, then you can rub any left over residue on those ashy knees or elbows.

Wonder Gro SHEA Butter

Mega Moisture Hairdress Conditioner

No-water base pomade. Great results. Modest price.

ALLWAYS 100% INDIAN HEMP

Naturally Medicated Herbal Hair & Scalp Treatment Conditioner

Great for Hand Grooming and No Comb hairstyles. It really tames virgin hair nicely. Great price - inexpensive.

HEAT SENSE by tcb

Recently tried, and was very pleased. Not expensive.

Gold Medal Hair Products Co.

1 Bennington Avenue,

Freeport, Long Island, New York 11520

Amazing mail-order catalog company which specializes in products designed for Black women who are maintaining natural "virgin" hair(chemical free). You will be very glad to be added to their mailing list.

Now, of course, I don't use all of these products all of the time. I mix it up according to style, my hair's needs, time, money, or availability of product. It's really liberating not

having to be dependent upon products made specifically for hair treated with chemicals. A few of the aforementioned products may not necessarily be appropriate for relaxed hair, but excellent for virgin hair. Have fun discovering the new world of hair products you can use for kinky, natural, woolly hairstyles.

"Look at me. I am Black. I am beautiful."

Mary McLeod Bethune

1875 - 1955

AUTHOR BIOGRAPHY

Ella Joyce, was born Cherron Hoye in Chicago, Illinois, and raised in Detroit, Michigan. After graduating from Cass Technical High School in the Performing Arts Curriculum, and attending the Dramatic Arts program at Eastern Michigan University, she worked as a legal secretary for fours years at Ford Motor Company, before deciding to pursue her love of acting as a career. She studied with several professional mentors and has worked many regional stages across America, and overseas. She is proud to be a regular attendee and performer at the **National Black Theater Festival** in Winston-Salem, North Carolina. She has received numerous awards, nominations, and accolades for her performances in theater, including the New York Audelco and the NAACP Image Nomination. In addition to landing the co-starring role of Eleanor on FOX TV's ***"Roc",*** she has appeared in many films such as New Line Cinema's, ***"Set It Off",*** Disney's ***"Selma, Lord Selma", "The Old Settler",*** HBO's ***"Stranger Inside", "Bubba Ho-Tep",*** TLC's award winning ***"Waterfalls"*** video, as well as guest appearances on televisions shows such as ***"Seinfeld", "The Client", "Jamie Foxx Show", "Dangerous Minds",*** and "***In The House",*** to name a few. She has graced the covers of many Black magazine publications including **JET**, **Black Elegance**, and **Black Masks**, and has been written up in **TV Times**. Ella also serves as a personal acting coach and consultant. Her representation is listed with Screen Actor's Guild (SAG), American Fedration of Television and Radio Artists (AFTRA), and Actor's Equity Association (AEA). This is Ella's first book.

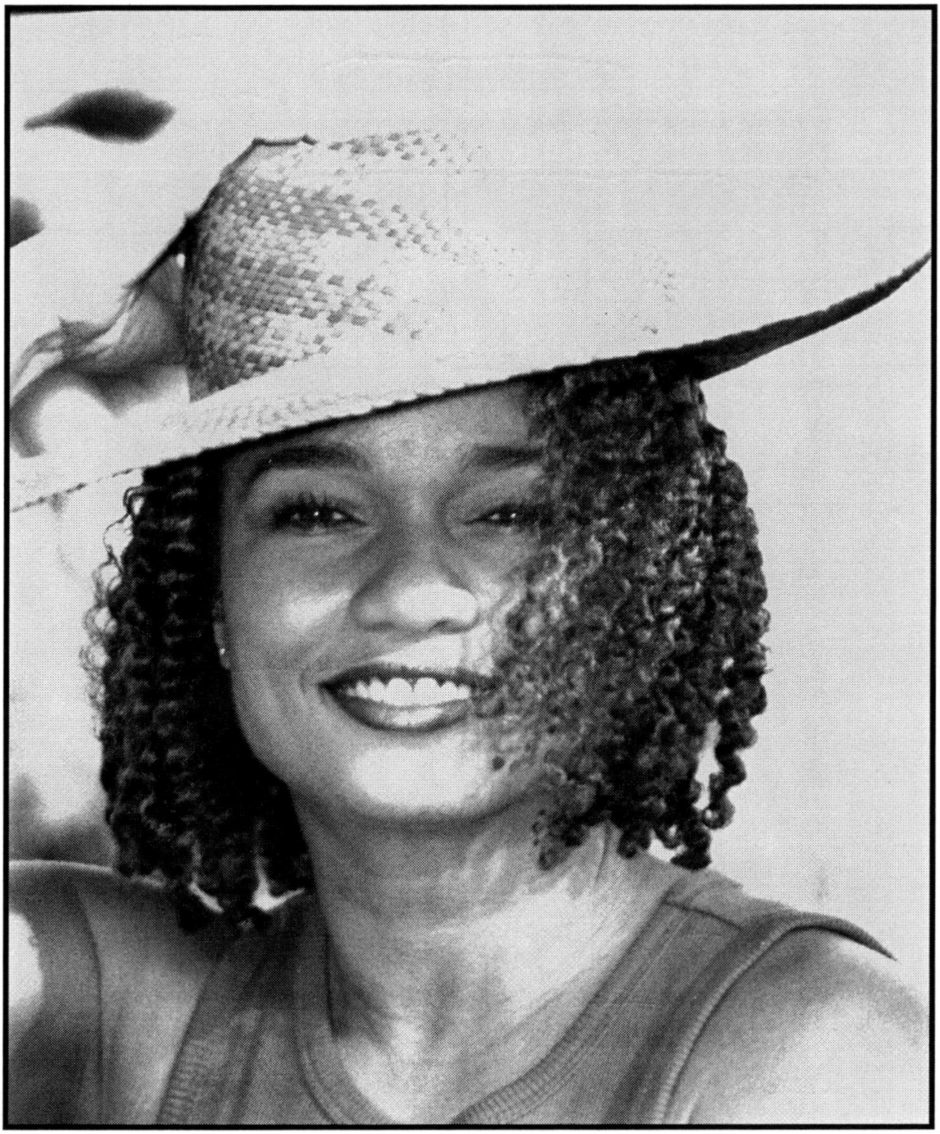

My first "bad hair" day

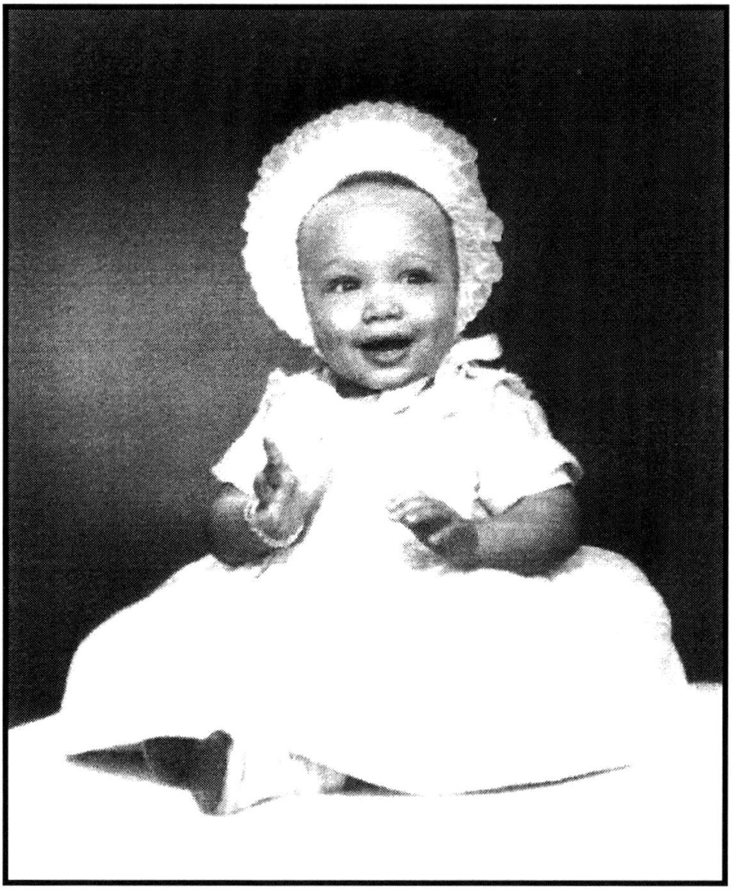

My Nana nicknamed me "Peaches" because of the peach-fuzz just beginning to grow from underneath my baby bonnet.

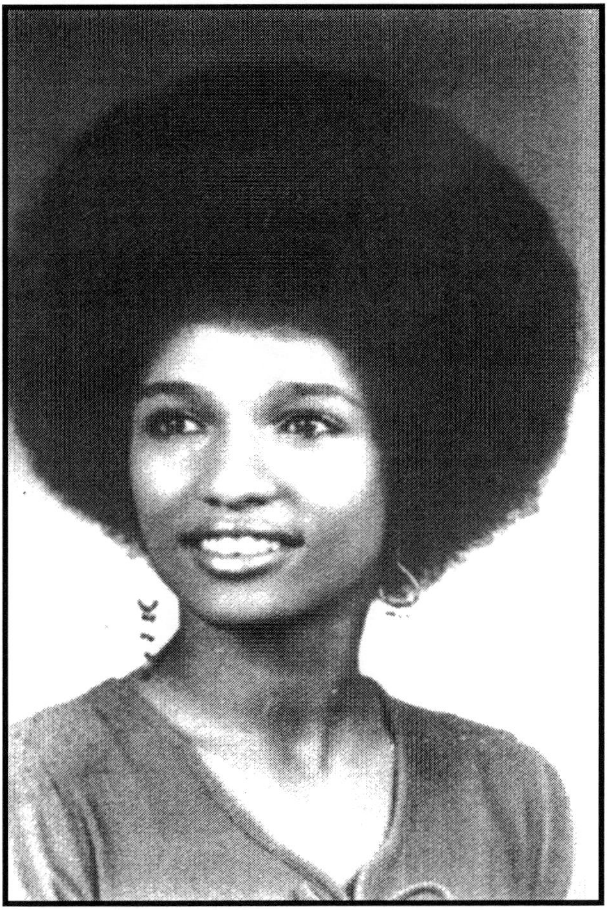

"Afro"

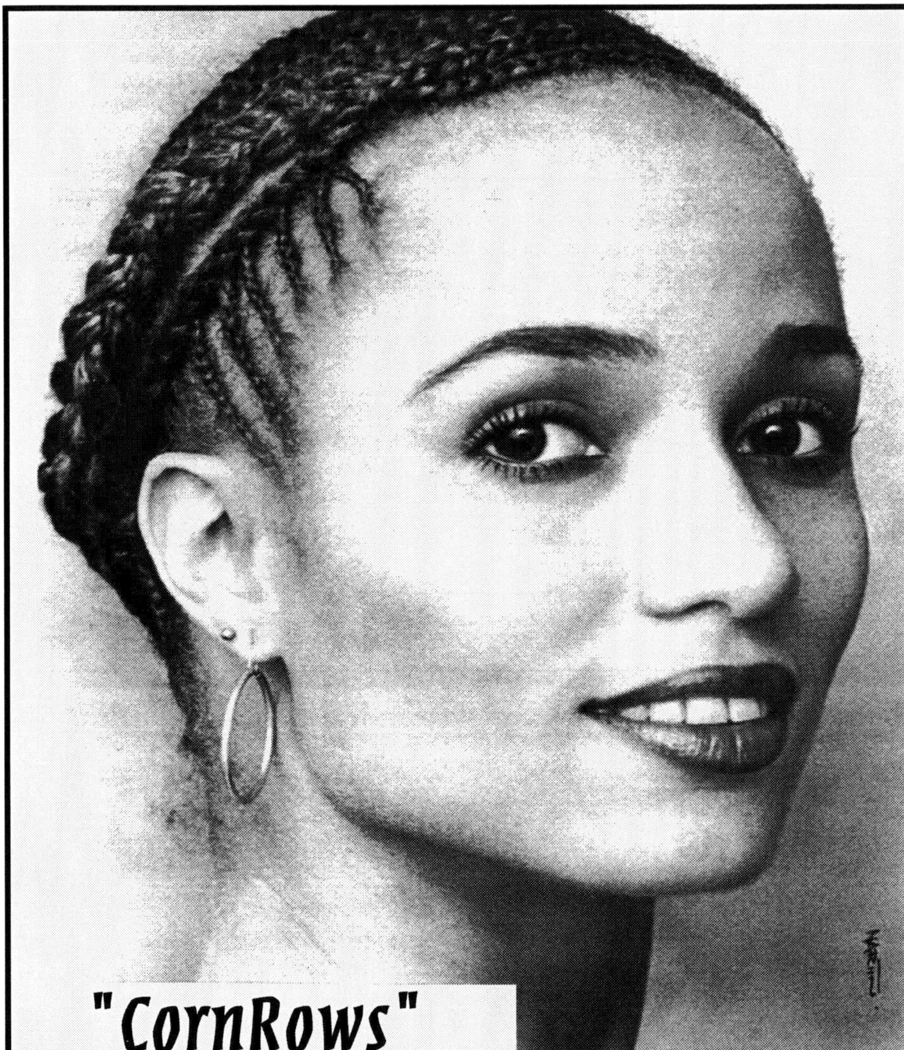

"CornRows"

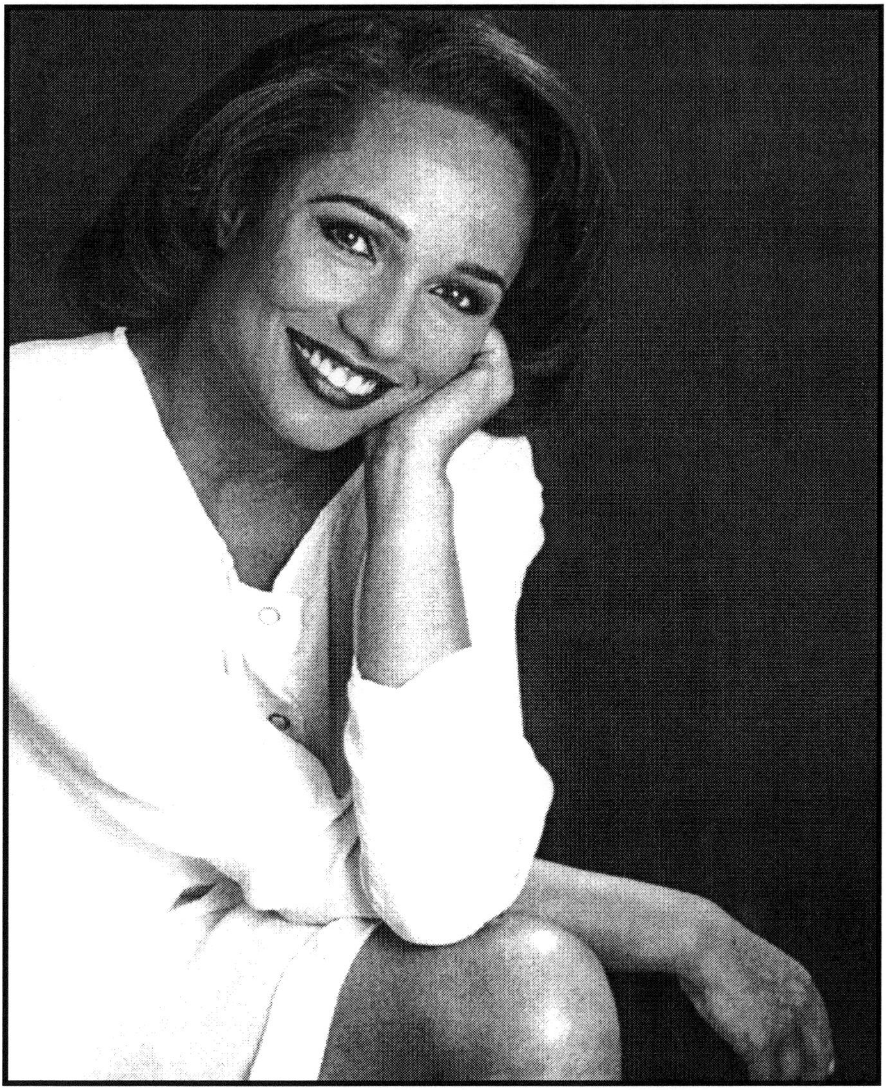

Of course, my hair was relaxed and hot curled for my role as "Eleanor" on the Fox sit-com "Roc". Relaxers are always beautiful, at first.

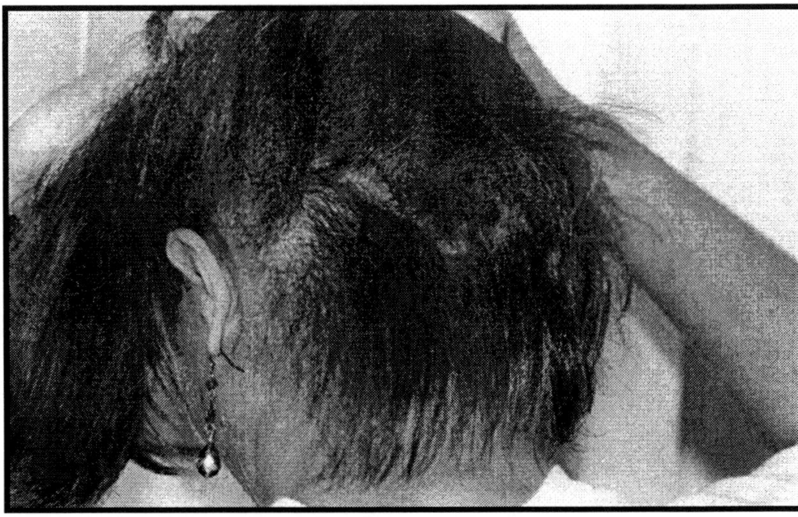

RIO destroyed my hair in the 90's

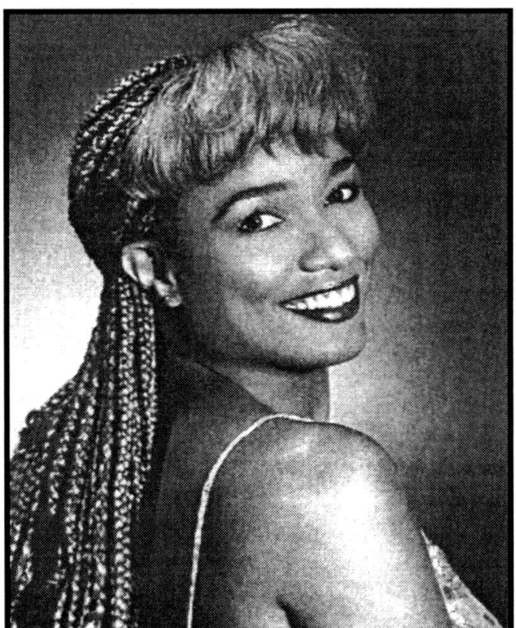

Life with braids. Light press n' curl bangs. My braider completedthis style in 4 hours straight, and the braids fell well past my waist.

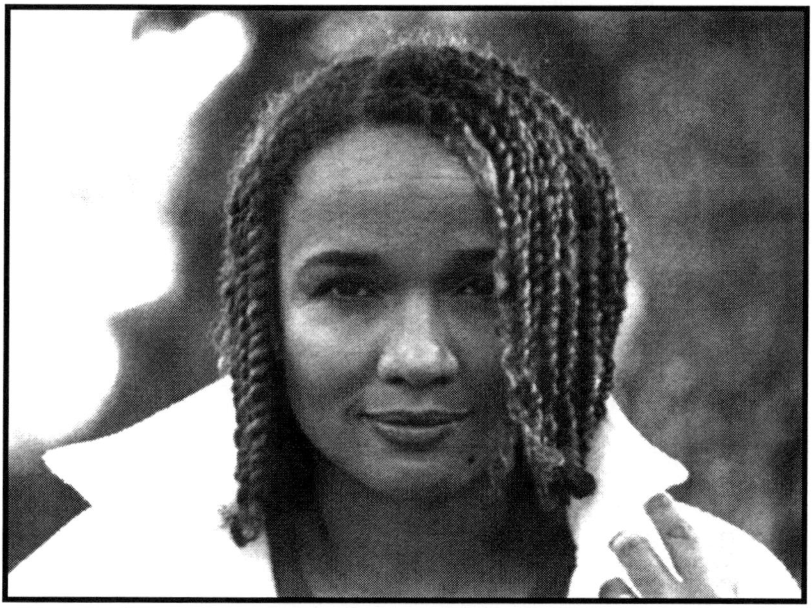

Right after shampooing and twisting hair, you can wear it that way without further styling if you choose. This is all of my own hair. It is still slightly damp, but I can go out in public.

Step One

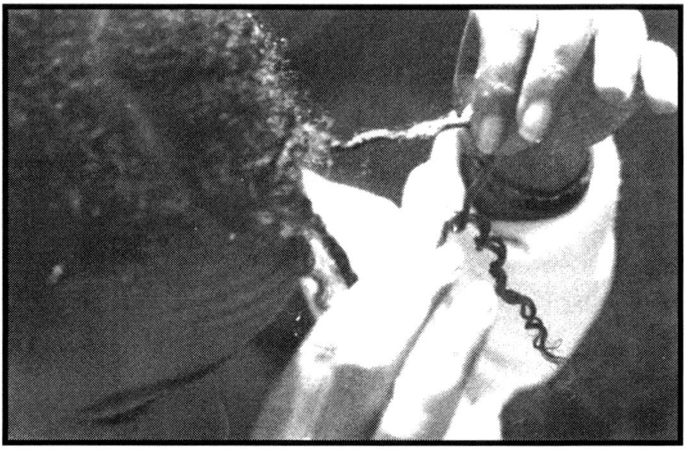

Start at the scalp when taking the Twists apart in one easy pull motion.

The curly waves will stay "set" if you don't comb them out to frizz.

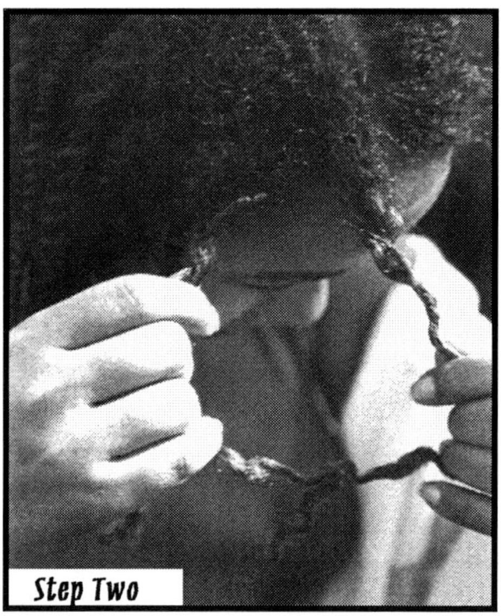

Step Two

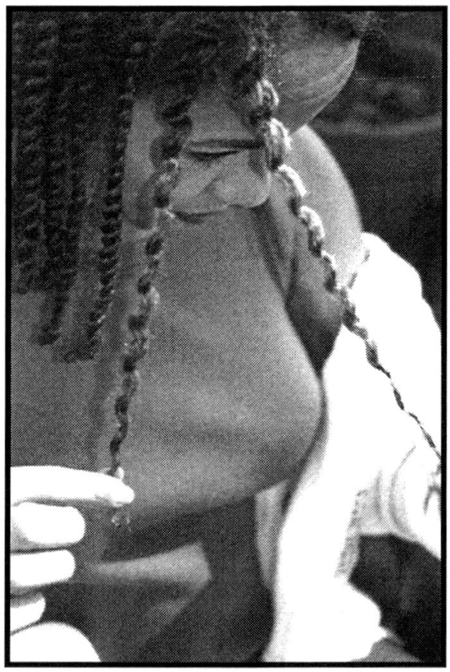

Step Three

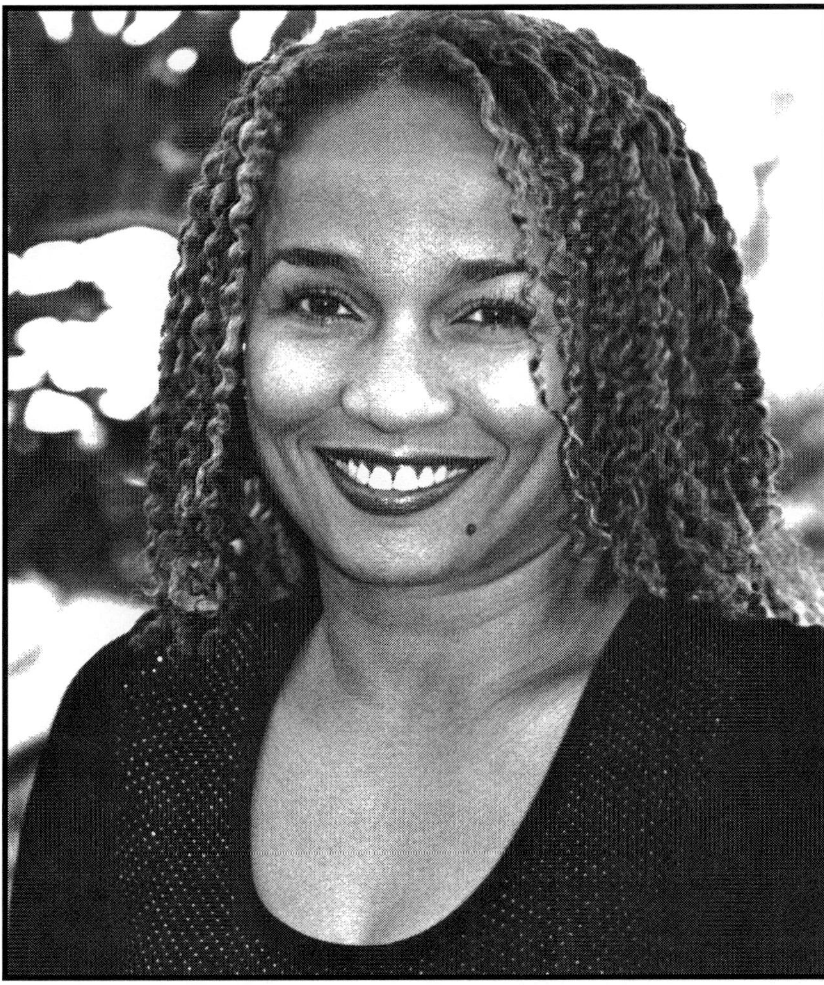

Ella's

"California Twists"

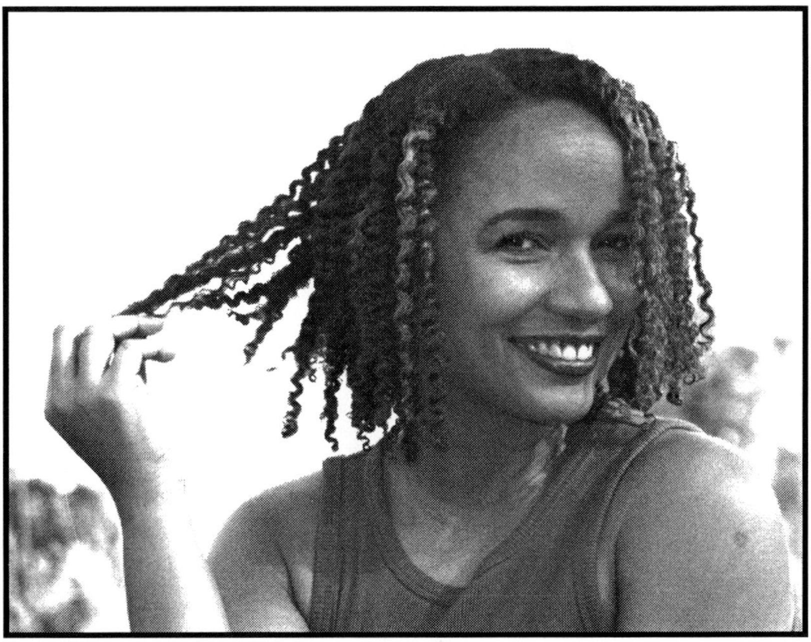

"No Comb"

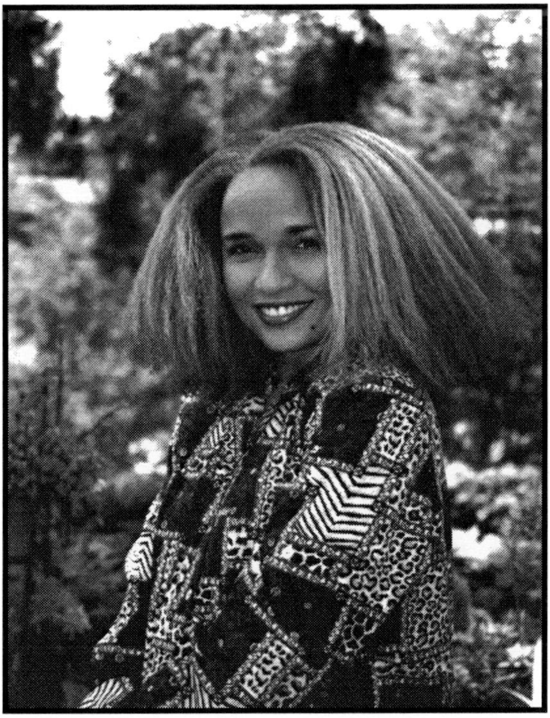

I lightly blow-dried my hair and ran a warm electric hotcomb through my hair for the first time in almost four years. I was shocked at how thick, long, and super soft my "virgin" hair was.

Note: If you fat-braid just the ends of this style with a gel you can achieve the hairstyle on the back cover of this book.

KINK PHOBIA

Journey Through A Black Woman's Hair

ORDER FORMS - retail paperback

Today's Date:____________________

Make check's payable to: First Publish, Inc.

First Publish, Inc.
300 Sunport Lane
Orlando, FL 32809
www.firstpublish.com

price: $12.95 each quantity______ (add 6% tax) Total:__________

method of payment: (Circle one) check cash credit card

Name (as appears on credit card): ______________________________

VISA # ____

Exp. date:____

Signature:(form not valid without signature for credit card purchase)

____

Shipping Address: ____________________________________

____

____

(Your copy will be sent directly from the printer. Please allow 3-4 weeks delivery.)

Thank you for you order!!